The
Healing Mission
and the
Business Ethic

Robert M. Cunningham, Jr.

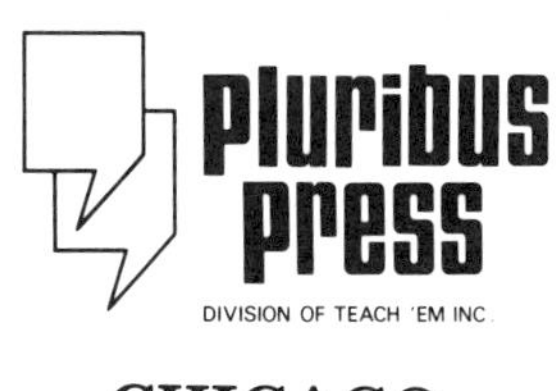

CHICAGO
1982

.Library of Congress Catalog Card Number:
81-84917

International Standard Book Number:
0-931028-21-3 (Clothbound)

Printed in the United States of America

Many of the articles in this collection were published originally in *Hospitals, J.A.H.A.,* copyright © 1977, 1978, 1979 by the American Hospital Association, and in *Hospitals* magazine, copyright © 1980, 1981 by American Hospital Publishing, Inc., and reprinted or adapted here by permission. Some others appeared initially in *Modern Hospital* and *Modern Healthcare,* copyright © 1969, 1972, 1973, 1974, 1975, 1976 by McGraw-Hill, Inc., and reprinted by permission.

PREFACE

As this is written, the Congress has just voted the three-year tax cut requested by the President, having approved his budget cuts a few weeks earlier. The President has told the striking air traffic controllers to get back to work or get fired, and all the voters who considered that government spending and the inflationary demands of labor had got out of hand and badly needed their comeuppance are applauding wildly—including many who are going to be hurt by the budget cuts and disarrangement of air travel. All over the country, editorial writers and columnists and commentators are busy writing pieces interpreting these events as further evidence of a profound shift in the national disposition. The era of liberal social thought introduced fifty years ago by President Franklin Roosevelt's New Deal has ended, they will say, and a new era of conservatism has begun— a return to reliance on private initiative as opposed to dependence on public support.

Given this environment, the outlook for the health care economy, and the health care system, is seen as conforming with the new social topography of the nation. Further increases in Medicare benefits are out of the question; instead, the effort will be to add deductibles and cut down unnecessary use of services. Cost reimbursement of providers will be discarded in favor of prospective payments offering incentives to hold costs down. Medicaid payments—state as well as federal—will be cut to the bone; choice by consumers will be restricted to selected low-cost providers. As soon as it can be managed, Medicare and Medicaid will both be switched to voucher systems that will require competing providers to toe the mark.

Widespread system reforms will follow the same course. Price competition among providers and insurers will be the prevailing mode; the efficient will prosper, those who can't make it will "be allowed to fail," in the curious locution of one of the enthusiasts for system reform. Competition is expected to make planning unnecessary, and the government planning apparatus conceived and developed over the past decade will be dismantled. It was expensive and ineffective, and, besides, the whole idea of planning is out of tune with the times. The unseen hand of competition, not the heavy hand of government, will guide development of the system. And the expectation is that with competition in the driver's seat the vagaries of insured fee-for-service practice in voluntary hospitals will give way to the efficiencies of health maintenance organizations and corporate hospital chains.

This is the way it looks to those who see the events of the past year as not merely a shift in the wind but a real sea change, as they like to say, a transformation of another order of magnitude. Whether it is one or the other will not be clear right away, and perhaps not for another decade or more. Either way, it will be plain to readers of the articles and essays in this volume that I am not wholly persuaded of the desirability of price competition as a guiding force for the delivery of medical services. Regulation as guide and control has been far from satisfactory, and at times oppressive, but scarcely to the point where the only solution is overthrow of the entire fee-for-service, health insurance, voluntary hospital establishment that for all its shortcomings has served most of the needs of the population so well for so many generations. To declare that most hospitals should become parts of for-profit marketing operations and that "hospitals going bankrupt . . . are the only answer to the overinvestment problem" sounds more like Marie Antoinette than what it actually was—the new federal budget director telling a conference about the administration's plans for the U.S. health care system.

The proposals for change, moderate as well as radical, the struggles with regulation, and other public issues that have engaged the attention of physicians, hospital executives, and trustees over the past decade, and especially the past three years, are all examined in these pages, along with considerations of patient care, institutional governance and management, and public opinion related to health care institutions and services. The pieces included here were written as the problems arose and the issues emerged, or as I perceived them to be arising and emerging, and they are presented here more nearly in accordance with the relevance of the subjects than with the timeliness or chronology of the events. Those who have lived through the past decade with hospital interests and responsibilities on their daily calendars won't have much trouble remembering what was going on as soon as the nature of each concern becomes clear. To give other readers, for whom these interests may be less urgent, some sense of direction, if not a road map, to help them find their way through the thicket of topical worries, the dates of original publication have been included in most cases, and explanatory notes have been added in some.

While it may be true that some of the problems I was writing about in 1973 and 1974, say, are not at the top of the lists on those hospital executive calendars today, there isn't anything here that is really irrelevant. Anybody who thinks that national health insurance is a dead issue because events now are moving in another direction, for example, need only be reminded that it has been considered a dead issue again and again over the past fifty years. It was a major worry, one way or another, of everybody in the health care field less than half a dozen years ago, and it will rise again from the dead in the 1980s as it did in the 1930s, and the 1940s, and the 50s and 60s and 70s. The same thing may be said about planning, and quality control, and hospital philanthropy, and all the other concerns that have been crowded off hospital calendars by the flap about regulation and competition. They'll all be back—and fee-for-service practice, and health insurance, and voluntary nonprofit hospitals, will still be around to cope with them.

The reason this can be said with assurance, at a time when the call to revolution is being heard, was explained thousands of years ago by King David: "I have been young and now am old," he said, "yet have I not seen the righteous forsaken." The cause of doctors and hospitals and health insurers is a righteous cause. It is caring for the sick and injured and making it as certain as can be done that the needs of the population for care will be met as they arise. The worry about cost and efficiency is real, and the effort to control cost and improve efficiency must go on, but to consider that health care is nothing more than an economic good to be marketed like every other good or service or commodity is to deny its essential quality that has endured for centuries and can't be shouted, or voted, out of existence.

Now anybody who goes out of his way to expose to public view another time the opinions he has expressed over a decade or more has to be either confident or crazy, because the likelihood that he has been right more than half the time is small, and nobody enjoys the embarrassment of appearing to lack either wit or wisdom. I am not especially confident of either the accuracy or the cogency of the opinions I have put down over the years as these are recorded again here, and I don't think I am crazy, at least not certifiably so. So readers of this book are certain to come across instances where I have been patently wrong, as readers have done right along when the pieces first appeared—on one memorable occasion causing an agitated lady to write the magazine's publisher that I had set back the progress of hospital volunteerism twenty-five years. But I have unshakable confidence in one opinion that appears consistently throughout these pages: The special quality of health care is something different from, and more than, and better than, an economic good. It is visible in the corridors of hospitals, if not always in the corridors of government, and it will endure for centuries more as it has for centuries past.

August 1981 —R.M.C., Jr.

CONTENTS

THE HEALING MISSION
AND THE BUSINESS ETHIC

THE HEALING MISSION AND THE BUSINESS ETHIC

The announcement early in 1981 that Hospital Corporation of America had acquired Hospital Affiliates International, formerly a property of the Insurance Company of North America, projected a $2 billion corporate giant in the hospital field and caused a flurry of excitement tinged with anxiety in the medical-hospital establishment, something like what the rest of the world might feel if Russia bought France and Germany. The new corporation would have five percent of all the beds and two percent of all the money, give or take, and that was enough to make a lot of people look around and say, "What's going on here?" The Institute of Medicine, which might be considered the House of Lords of a class-conscious profession, invited a group of heavy thinkers to a meeting in Washington to examine the impact of corporate interest in medical affairs, where it turned out that Arnold Relman of the *New England Journal of Medicine* regarded the rise of corporate activity as a menace on the way to being a disaster, and Mike Bromberg of the Federation of American Hospitals considered the same phenomenon as a fulfillment of the American Dream. Some like it hot and some like it cold. A leading hospital consultant put out a position paper urging the organization of "doctor corporations" to defend the profession against eventual domination by powerful outsiders, but it wasn't clear what the corporations were expected to do. A few wiseacres who have been predicting for the past 10 years that the corporate chains would become the dominant force in the hospital field saw the HCA-HAI merger as evidence that they had been right all along, and some leaders of the traditional hospital culture whose positions and institutions are obviously secure insisted that the corporate onslaught is simply an element of the free market that you have to favor if you believe in free enterprise—an argument that is embarrassed by Section 7 of the Clayton Act prohibiting activities that can have the effect of diminishing competition. The Clayton Act was passed by the Congress in 1914 and remains something less than a sensational success in prohibiting activities that can have the effect of diminishing competition, possibly because the prohibited activities were not very clearly defined in the first place and not made any clearer by the Supreme Court decision in the U.S. Steel case in 1920 declaring that "the law does not make mere size an offense."

Mere size is not an offense according to law, but size can be a problem in human affairs. Size, for example, has been one of our principal complaints against government. Big government is equated with bad government; this is the assumption that has given rise to the block grant movement, which postulates that state and local management is superior to federal jurisdiction. The proposition has an attractive logic, but in practice it is likely to prove disappointing: The units are smaller but not necessarily more manageable; given the nature of politicians and bureaucrats, the state and local varieties are not always more competent or more amenable to reason than the federal species. More often than not, the reverse proves to be the case.

The feeling about big government is unique. In everything else, it is the disposition of the society to consider large size a virtue *per se*. This is most notably true in the case of business and industry, where big is good and bigger is better. The Fortune Five Hundred are the nation's acknowledged corporate elite, set apart by size alone. Board chairmen announce proudly at the annual meeting of shareholders that last year's performance elevated the company from 278th place on the list to 275th, an obvious cause for rejoicing. A proposed merger of E.I. duPont and Conoco evokes black headlines and breathless leads; if approved, the combination would create a *thirty billion dollar company*! Wherever you are, Senator Clayton, how do you like *that*?

The values in business are seen as the antithesis of values in government. The assumption in business is that greatness resides at national headquarters; local and regional managers are lesser types. Branch managers who succeed advance to the region, and thence to valhalla. Nobody stops to consider that the U.S. senator who started his political life as a state assemblyman and the Washington bureau chief who began as a park commissioner in Wauwatosa have climbed the same ladder as the board chairman who used to be a salesman in Buffalo, so the block grants make about as much sense as it would to turn the corporate budget over to the accountant in Crystal Falls. Big is good in business and big is bad in government. That's the way it is, and that's the way it is going to stay.

The uneasiness about the HCA-HAI hospital corporation merger suggests that value judgments in the hospital field do not conform wholly to the business system, though certainly they lean that way. Inevitably, the larger the hospital, the better its services are commonly judged to be, not only in breadth or scope, which is likely to be true, but also in quality, which may or may not be. Similarly, though to a lesser extent, the same values are sometimes ascribed to the profession. But "the bigger the practice the better the doctor" is a wrong standard wherever it may be applied. A single example will show why: "The doctor I worked with at the clinic where I took my OB clinical prided himself on the numbers of patients he could see every day," an observant nurse said in a recent interview on medical and nursing values. "'Oh, sixty patients today? Well, yesterday I did sixty-nine.' He was like that. He was slick. Very politically aware. If he had some important person in there, he'd spend extra time. He would give me the clinic patients, the ones with the green cards. But the thing that absolutely horrified me in that experience was that I never saw that doctor wash his hands between patients. Not once in three months. His emphasis was on numbers, and efficiency. He was very efficient. He'd talk on the phone and look in the microscope at the same time. He was one of those people who could do five things at once. You really have to spell things out for people, and that hurried attitude discourages patients from feeling free to ask."

For all that, the doctor had a good reputation and a huge practice, the nurse reported—evidence enough that a lot of people are using the business standard to judge professional value.

Doctors have better standards for judging one another, but some of these are less reliable than others. Thus according to one yardstick in common use a graduate of Harvard Medical School is presumed to be a better doctor than, say, a graduate of the University of Alabama College of Medicine, though this may not be true in any particular case, and the proposition would be certain to start an argument almost anywhere in the South. Besides, the reach and complexity of medicine is such that comparisons are questionable to begin with; the Harvard man might know more about molecular biology while the Alabaman could take better care of a stroke patient. So who is to say which is the better doctor? Better for what? And wherever he came from, the doctor who brags about seeing 69 patients a day and forgets to wash his hands is a bad risk for all of them.

Most specialists have their own method of assessing competence among their peers. The head of otolaryngology may not know beans about an obstetrician or an internist at his own place, but ask him about an otolaryngologist in Pittsburgh or Butte, and he'll get a reliable professional reading in about three phone calls. "Who'd he train with?" he'll want to know, and when he gets the name of the chief of service where the unknown doctor spent his residency, he can quickly find someone who has all the answers. In their three or four or more years of residency training, young physicians reveal all their strengths and weaknesses to their teachers; often they take on the character and mannerisms, as well as the professional methods and skills, of the chief. "If he trained with so-and-so, he's all right," physicians often say with confidence of someone they never heard of before but whose teacher is well known. It's a professional variation of the Old Boys' Network, and it includes an element of professional snobbery, but it works. He probably wouldn't say so to anybody but a trusted colleague, but the chances are that the OB chief at the place where the slick doctor who didn't wash his hands had his residency knew all about the student's habits. "Smart as a whip," he'd say. "But you gotta watch him. He cuts corners."

Cutting corners is medicine's major sin, according to the late Walsh McDermott, M.D., distinguished professor of medicine at

Cornell University, editor of a textbook of medicine that is in use throughout the world, and one of the profession's most revered teachers. "The major sins, perhaps the greatest, are those sins of omission wherein the physician cuts a corner and because of fatigue, laziness, or sense of time pressure, fails to perform some examination or obtain some test, and as a result of the omission some patient has been harmed," Dr. McDermott wrote recently. "What we mean when we say that a person is a good physician is that the person can be trusted. As one cannot reasonably be expected never to make a mistake, by 'trusted' is meant that there is a high degree of probability that this physician will provide care of high quality in a determinable set of circumstances. In short, an all-important self-discipline is present. The great vital principle—the secret, if you will, of medical education and training at its highest quality—lies not in impressive facilities or glittering diagnostic apparatus, but in this deep-seated tradition of self-discipline. For unlike the development of skills in other learned professions, the part of medicine that has to do with the clinical examination of the patient yields an almost exact return for the effort put into it. The key is thoroughness, invariable thoroughness, and as the affair is usually conducted in private, there is no one to monitor the physician's thoroughness. Well aware of this fact, and aware that the probabilities are such that one could get away with time-saving omissions without discovery—at least in the short run, the physician must have been so deeply convinced that he or she bears an inviolable responsibility for thoroughness that any lapse is the equivalent of a conscious, harmful act to someone given into his or her trust.

"This is what one cannot see simply by watching another physician's acts—this meticulousness, the sense of always exploring every nook and cranny of the problem. This acquisition of the deep conviction of the essentiality of thoroughness is the most important feature of the education given in a medical school. By long tradition, the physicians who carry the major responsibility for clinical teaching have this attribute, and they spend much of their time imprinting it in the students. . . . I emphasize the point that this quality is invisible, and there is really no way it can be determined except by observation of the student or physician in action over a considerable period of time. This is what is done in the last two years of medical school and also in the several years of residency. It is on the basis of such observation that the faculty or the hospital attending staff can say that someone is a good doctor. As physicians cannot do this when they meet a strange physician, they do the next best thing—they set great store by where that physician received education and training."[1]

Plainly "more is better" as a standard works well in medicine when it means more care for the individual patient—not necessarily more services, but more care by doctors and nurses taking pains to make certain they understand all the dimensions of the illness or injury of *this patient* and are doing all they know how to do, and getting all the help they need, to make this patient well. This is also the mission of the hospital as an institution of healing, but this kind of "more is better" medicine is not always consonant with the "more is better" purpose of the hospital as an institution of business. During the years when hospitals were growing along with the population, industry, the medical profession, and the health insurance system, the healing mission and the "more is better" business ethic got along together comfortably enough for the most part, though there were always stressful times when the doctors' demands for new equipment and special personnel collided with the administrators' judgment of what might be considered prudent investments. But as third parties became the dominant sources of revenue, and payors became more and more concerned about just what services they were paying for, pressures on management to control spending mounted, and the paths of the healing mission and the business ethic diverged sharply at times. Throughout the inflationary years of the past decade, the pressures have been relentless; the healing mission and the business ethic often go in opposite directions, yet the hospital must respond to both imperatives.

Even during these years, however, it has generally been possible for trustees, managers, and physicians to work out reasonable accommodations of the countervailing imperatives without seriously damaging either the quality of patient care or the stability of institutional operations. But it is never easy to do, and it is getting harder all the time. And whether one considers that the deregulation emphasis and free competition proposals of the new federal administration promise liberation and opportunity for hospitals and doctors, as many do, or will simply substitute one set of pressures for another, as some insist, the dichotomy of purpose seems certain to continue, and it could get worse. Whether the pressure on spending comes from regulatory authority or competitive enterprise, the hospital must continue to attend both healing mission and business ethic, and whether the pressure comes from self-discipline or partnership or group practice or hospital, the physician will continue to owe a duty of diligence to both his patients and his economic environment. For both hospital and physician, the balancing act will go on.

The conflicting pressures exist in all institutions and all practices, but they are not totally unrelated to size. It is obviously unwise to generalize in the absence of specific information, but it would appear that accommodating the need of patients for care and the need of managers for money must be easier in small institutions and small communities, where the people on both sides see each other every day, than it can be in larger institutions where the needs of patients are monitored by one hierarchy and the needs of managers by another, and communications are filtered through committees. And considering the rule that says, "the likelihood that the decision at the margin will favor the patient care instead of the economy alternative varies inversely with the distance from the bedside," it isn't surprising that it is in the larger hospitals and systems that the balance seems to be tipping more often toward business purpose. It isn't that anybody wants it or wills it that way; it is simply that this is where the pressures are heaviest and most visible. The cost figures are all in Macy's window, but nobody may notice when a medication or treatment is missed because it was an aide and not a nurse who was responsible for the schedule, or because the unit was understaffed, or because the doctor was too busy to check. In small places, moreover, there isn't anybody around who can say "Now wait just a minute" to a doctor; in big places these people are all over.

This is not to suggest the absurd—that patient care is better in small hospitals than it is in large hospitals. The odds go the other way, for obvious reasons of staff talent, professional and technical personnel, equipment, facilities, and money. But bed for bed and dollar for dollar, the small place may make a better show of holding the healing mission line against the business infiltration.

Actually, nobody is trying to "hold the line." What line? There is no conscious recognition of divergent aims. Ask any physician, any trustee, any executive, about the mission of the hospital, and you're going to get an answer something like, "to take the best possible care of patients at the lowest possible cost," with no thought that this is a purpose that at times must argue with itself. Ask about the hospital's plans for the future, and except in the rarest of cases the answer now is going to comprehend growth—the addition of new services to keep in step with advances in medicine, certainly, and with few exceptions also some growth in size, even in communities where the population is static, because 125 beds beats 100, for the same reason that 600 is better than 500. Even in medicine, you can't get completely away from the Fortune Five Hundred paradigm.

A new resource that has been developing rapidly in the past decade to help hospitals cope with business pressures could either assist or complicate the accommodation of healing mission and business ethic. This is the multi-hospital organization, which had been around for years in the form of loose shared-service arrangements and common ownership or affiliation with religious orders. The advent of corporate chains in the early Medicare and Medicaid years was at first brushed off by the traditional hospital field as inconsequential, but when the chains moved aggressively to build, acquire, and make contracts to manage more hospitals, and more substantial hospitals, it became apparent that the original judgment had been in error. Then, as the complexities of the Economic Stabilization Program, the Planning Act, PSRO, the Hill-Burton charitable requirement, changing third party payments, Medicare and Medicaid, rising malpractice liability, the Cost of Living Council, raging inflation, and a few other amenities affecting hospital business office practice began to pile up and tax the capacity and sanity of the individual hospital executive, the appeal of coalition became increasingly attractive. The movement of independent hospitals into management systems has been for the most part a defensive maneuver—not just against the corporate chains but against the adversities and misadventures of institutional life in a regulated society.

As gospel emerges from teaching and then teaching from gospel, so the literature of a business or profession emerges first from action of some kind, followed by action based on the literature. Thus the early multi-hospital systems created a substantial volume of research papers and journal articles, which are now being used by boards of trustees and executives as the basis for decisions about multi-hospital systems. There is no hard and fast agreement yet about what a multi-hospital system *is*, actually, but several different types have been identified and according to one of the recognized scholars of these phenomena, the general classifications are: (1) affiliations, or combinations among institutions designed for specific and limited joint undertakings; (2) management contracts, with the hospital retaining its separate identity and governing authority and the contractor responsible for operations within defined limits; (3) the separate or "umbrella" corporation that performs either limited or full management functions for one or several hospitals, and (4) merger or consolidation, with separate hospitals becoming a single corporate entity.[2]

These and other multi-hospital arrangements are commonly justified on the ground of efficiencies to be gained through economies of scale. "Classical economic arguments are invoked that a larger organization can better use expensive equipment, obtain volume purchases, capture the advantages of specialization, and obtain capital at lower cost," said David B. Starkweather, Ph.D., professor of health administration at the University of California School of Public Health in Berkeley. But, he warned, "research suggests that there is an initial period of inefficiency. Unit costs are higher than they would be without merger. This period of initial inefficiency can easily last for eight to twelve years."[3]

Eight to twelve years of inefficiency might appear to be a high price to pay for shelter from the vagaries of external circumstance, but Dr. Starkweather considers that there are other gains. "In general, merged hospital systems improve the quality of care," he said. "This occurs because the reorganizations force the examination of previously unsupervised activities and often yield new forms of quality audit and control. In addition, there is the quality gain that goes along with size or volume: i.e., open-heart surgeries are conducted where there is sufficient volume to provide practice and expertise for the surgical and nursing teams. These improvements in quality come with at least commensurate increases in cost. Further, multi-hospital arrangements usually lead to a broader scope of services available to a community or an area."

Commenting further on the effects of hospital systems, Dr. Starkweather noted that the new arrangement usually results in shifts in the balance of power within the hospital. Local trustees are likely to experience a decline in influence, either because a new board at a higher corporate level takes on some policy functions, or because "managements usually experience increased influence because of the complexity of the arrangement, which naturally brings to center stage the full-time administrative personnel who have the knowledge and commitment to see things through." Doctors, on the other hand, may lose influence, "because their traditional dominance of local hospital affairs is often replaced by a more remote management and governance less responsive to the doctors' informal power."

Whether the rise of the multi-hospital arrangement will tilt events in favor of the healing mission or the business ethic at points where these are opposing causes must remain for resolution in specific institutions, and perhaps from day to day within institutions. Where the quality of care is improved by the addition of professional resources without notable attrition due to declining doctor power and added remoteness of governing authority, the healing mission may be enhanced, or at least protected. But where no great gains in services result and communication is attenuated by added size, distance, and complexity, the balance could be expected to shift toward the business ethic. And of course there are systems, as well as institutions, where the tension of conflicting imperatives is under control and the business ethic supports the healing mission instead of threatening it. But there are more hospital executives who insist that this is the case in their institutions than there are institutions in which it really is.

Even in places where the tension is under control, it could easily come undone in the competitive era in medical care we are headed into as fast as the Congress can put together a new law to get us there. As proposed, and applauded on all sides by (a) those who believe it promises freedom from regulation and (b) those who doubt that it does anything of the kind but figure any change has to be an improvement, the new law will require employers to offer their employees a choice of all the health plans in sight, and make the same contributions to all of them. Employers, it is expected, will then shop around among doctors and hospitals and choose the least expensive plans, and employees, who up to now when there has been a choice generally have chosen the more comprehensive, and more expensive, plans, will change their habits and opt for less expensive ones, to keep from spending their own money.

This free market or consumer's choice system is needed to give doctors and hospitals, as well as consumers, incentives to save instead of the incentive to spend that is encouraged by the present fee-for-service, cost reimbursement health insurance system, proponents of the new law insist. They either don't acknowledge or deny that it might also have the effect of encouraging doctors to see 69 patients a day and skip such inefficient wastes of time as hand-washing—an eventuality feared by some critics of the proposed law. Invisible but time-consuming virtues like Dr. McDermott's self-discipline do not rate high scores on the value scale of the economists and budget directors who are master-minding the advent of price competition in medical care. Inviolable responsibility for thoroughness? Exploring every nook and cranny of the problem? If you can't put it in the computer and put a price on it, and market it, forget it!

The extent to which the business ethic is ascendant in the world of hospitals and doctors is demonstrated in the changing terminology of the professional culture, whose mystique is evaporating rapidly—especially among hospital executives, who consider that "hospital industry" has a more authoritative resonance than "hospital field," and for whom "marketing the hospital's services" is what they do. "Meeting the community's needs," as their predecessors did, was all right for its time but, you know, *wishy-washy*. Whatever it's called, the process is one of defining the population to be served, assessing its needs for services within an institution's capabilities, preparing to deliver the services, and making certain the population is aware of their availability.

Many hospital governing boards, executives, and physicians were performing these tasks a generation ago, using the techniques that were generally available, and in some cases borrowing data from the public utility companies that were leaders in making population projections. Hospitals called it planning, and a lot of it was related to expansion of facilities, and except in small, remote communities it was all competitive. It wasn't until the 1970s, actually, when years of talk about a putative doctor shortage had doubled and then tripled the production of physicians and the shortage had become a surplus, and years of new hospitals and additions had created excesses of buildings and beds, and Medicare and Medicaid had made these public problems because public money was involved, that government regulations to curb the excesses and the competition were laid on and refinements of the planning process were borrowed increasingly from industry, which called it marketing. For the past three or four years, at least, the marketing effort has been focused principally on filling empty beds and finding new sources of revenue, and doing both these things ahead of the competition. These are business goals, not necessarily relevant to the healing mission except as they may add or subtract pressures on doctors to save money.

It isn't clear yet what the addition of price competition is going to do to this complex of forces. It may have the desirable effect of controlling spending, or it may not make that much difference, and it may have the undesirable effect of discouraging the inviolable thoroughness of good doctors, or it may not make that much difference here either. But in any case it seems certain to accelerate and expand hospital use of marketing techniques by adding another set of values to the competitive scramble, and that is either good or bad, depending on where you sit. It is good for all the marketing executives and consultants in hospitals, certainly, giving them another instrument for the brass sections of their orchestras; and it is good for the governing boards and chief executives of hospitals, with new data for their computers and new reach and precision for their projections; and good for employers and health plans that learn to play the new game and look around for the bargains in health care, and good for the employees and their families and others in the population who want to or have to look for bargains and are lucky enough to find those that are made possible by real efficiencies and not by cutting corners. But it is bad for good doctors whose invisible self-discipline instructs them to "perform some examination or obtain some test" that over time could result in price disadvantages for their institutions or health plans; and bad for the governing boards and chief executives who applaud their physicians' inviolable thoroughness and lose business in the price farrago as a consequence; and bad for the employers and employees and their families and others in the population who aren't lucky at all and end up choosing the bargains in health plans and hospitals whose governing boards and chief executives either don't know or don't care about the invisible self-discipline of good doctors and whose doctors, or some of them, don't wash their hands.

It should be understood that the good things and the bad things are not all going to be turned loose by some new law on competition and some new surge of interest in marketing. All these forces have been there right along; the tension between the healing mission and the business ethic is nothing new. In fact, it was the long-standing tendency of hospital governing boards and executives and physicians to use the healing mission as a screen to hide or excuse bad business practice that permitted many of the excesses of the decades of expansion to develop and made the rise of the business ethic in hospitals necessary and inevitable, along with the rise of the profit corporations and the rise of regulation. For most of the past decade, the pendulum has been swinging the other way, and the need now is to keep the business drive from gaining the upper hand to the point of suppressing the healing mission.

As long as the healing mission (and the concept of healing can readily be broadened to include activities directed toward prevention of disease and injury, and, as we say now, toward wellness) remains the central focus, it doesn't matter that much, or at least is not necessarily a cause for alarm, if the enterprise is a for-profit corporation instead of a traditional non-profit organization—or, as a growing number of hospitals and systems are, a combination of both. Hospitals and systems of all kinds must earn profits, or surpluses of revenue over expense, in order to survive. Disposition of the surplus—to investors as a return on the capital they have provided, in the one case, and directly into capital of one kind or another, in the other—is the technical difference. If there is also an underlying philosophic difference, as traditional hospital people would have insisted was the case 20 years ago, and many still do, it has been diminishing over the years and has largely vanished with the rise of the business ethic during the period of financial and regulatory pressures. Whatever the form of organization, it is still possible for the hospital to have the kind of business practice that supports the healing mission without the kind of "more is better" business ethic that threatens it, remembering that the former, and not the latter, is the purpose of the enterprise.

Whether we have more such hospitals in the future than we've had in the past will be determined not by law, nor by the articles of incorporation, but by the behavior of the principal actors.

[1]McDermott, Walsh, Educating Physicians for the Future, in McNerney, Walter J., Working for a Healthier America. Cambridge, MA: Ballinger Publishing Company, 1980.

[2]Starkweather, David B., Trends and Types of Multi-Hospital Arrangements. Technical Assistance Memo 56. San Francisco: Western Center for Health Planning, 1980.

[3]Starkweather, David B., The Pros and Cons of Multi-Hospital Systems. Technical Assistance Memo 57. San Francisco: Western Center for Health Planning, 1980.

THIS IS WHERE WE CAME IN

You Can't Rationalize
This Industry

A dozen years ago health care was six percent of GNP and the worry was too few doctors, not too many, but the values and the viewpoints weren't all that different.

January 1969

The hospital field is scrutiny-prone, and over the years it has suffered a parade of anthropologists, sociologists, economists, educators, engineers, mathematicians, and public administrators, among others, to promenade through its corridors, pointing and rolling eyes toward the ceiling. More often than not, these invasions have been initiated by hospital people themselves, whose capacity to absorb punishment is matched only by the eagerness of the nonhospital world to lay it on. Periodically, for example, hospital groups have invited representatives from other disciplines to sit down with them and examine hospital phenomena, an exercise that is frequently instructive on both sides but may have some of the characteristics, and some of the effects, of an icy shower, with one group pouring on cold water and the other bobbing and weaving and gasping for breath.

This was what could have been anticipated last month when the American College of Hospital Administrators invited a small group of economists, sociologists and others to come to Chicago for a day and a half of conversation about the value system in health affairs. Predictably, the occasion at times had one group laying the lash on hospitals and the other defending the health system. Unpredictably and uniquely in this case, however, it was the hospital people who did most of the criticizing and the economists who insisted things aren't really that bad. To be sure, this switching of roles came about near the end of the discussion and was preceded by several hours of talk that followed more accustomed paths, and it was only when the economists fell to brooding about the essential illogic of hospitals planning to cut down hospital beds, as they are being urged to do, that the turnaround occurred. "The hospital industry has rather uncritically accepted a characterization of itself as inefficient and disorderly, but it may be very orderly," a professor of economics declared suddenly. "The kinds of pressure you're subjected to make this understandable, but you're too defensive. I think you need competition in this industry, and you're always going to have some excess capacity lying around. But an inappropriate short-run solution such as cutting down the number of beds may make it harder for you to find rational solutions for the long run."

Unlike members of the House Ways and Means Committee, whose breathing becomes labored as they consider that the Social Security Administration may be paying millions for hospital care that could be given for one-third as much, or less than that, in nursing homes or outpatient departments, the economists contemplated this possibility without panic and suggested that the supply of physicians obviously needed to be increased, and it might not be a bad idea to increase the supply of beds, too, as long as the physician and patient always had a range of options or modalities of care from which to choose. The thing to do, they suggested, is to get rid of the irregularities that clog the system, such as insurance that creates incentives for hospital use and rationing imposed by organized medicine. "Much of the concern about cost and price stems from apprehension about the structure of the market," said the professor. "Clean up the structure, and you'd eliminate a lot of the discontent. Six per cent (of gross national product) might not be too high a price for health services, if we didn't have to worry about efficiency. And let's stop talking about 'overutilization.' We incorporate our decisions in our terminology! We should say 'appropriate utilization'."

Much as they liked this kind of talk, hospital administrators in the group were not especially comforted by it, because many of the them feel it is too late to learn the choreography of market concepts in the health system. The Congress, and perhaps the public, are already assuming the public facility status of hospitals and will no longer permit the free play of competition among health services, even if it were known to contribute to efficiency. Regulation is here, an administrator said; price controls loom.

The preceding discussion had briefly considered the possibility that, contrary to what most economists and hospital administrators have always thought, the health system is indeed a market that can be rationalized, like the market for red shoes or green peas. Prices decrease as the quantity produced exceeds demand, the market dictum goes, then demand quickens with falling price, and new supply is created as a response to the added, or newly visible, demand. But it doesn't work that way in the health field at all, the hospital people insisted; in fact, it is just the other way around. Here demand is comparatively unrelated to price, and demand responds to supply, instead of *vice versa*: Beds that are built will be occupied, the hospital aphorism has it.

The economists didn't believe it. "If supply really increases demand we're in real trouble," one of them said. "If this is true, it's next to impossible to rationalize this industry." Another postulated that the health service market does in effect follow the normal cycle, because demand here emerges from some form of physician-consumer interaction and it can be argued that when beds are freely available the convenience of use is equivalent to a falling price that evokes increased demand, with an ensuing supply response. This seemed a doubtful proposition to the hospital group, who were also unimpressed by an economist's suggestion that the way to bring health costs down is to increase the supply, or number, of physicians, thereby intensifying competition. Physicians would reduce their fees, the argument ran, and try to find ways to save their patients money, such as using less expensive alternatives for hospital care.

Something like this might conceivably happen, it was acknowledged, if it were possible to double the number of physicians overnight, thus flooding the market for their services. Short of this, the effect of the gradually increasing number of physicians is simply added utilization, and added cost, and prices keep right on climbing anyway. The prospect isn't notably promising for hospitals under public attack and threats of public control, but the economists seemed cheered to have hit upon something that made sense, at least theoretically, out of the health system.

In addition to the hospital administrators and economists,

the colloquium, as it was elegantly titled, included two sociologists, a political scientist, and a professor of health service administration. Members who didn't fit precisely into either the hospital or academic classifications included an urban university executive who masterminds his institution's involvement in neighborhood activities, the director of a conference of church hospitals, and a health service prepayment administrator with flawless credentials as a thinker and lecturer on health service systems. The collective assignment was to search out values in health affairs, and the assumption was that examination of the value system would somehow aid in making judgments about "not only what to do and how to do it but also when to do it and why."

Identification and definition of values presented no great difficulty, but ordering them so as to bear in shaping decisions proved another matter altogether; here the discussion quickly encountered a thicket of complexities. Sanctity of life and tender, loving care were instantly accepted as values, for example; so were technical skill and the over-all efficiency of the health service. But technical skill may often shred tender, loving care beyond all recognition, and over-all efficiency may be diluted, if not destroyed, when enormous concentrations of resources are required to prolong lives that age and disease have rendered all but meaningless. Caught up in such contradictions, the discussion began to fibrillate, and on occasion it turned out that the consensus on values was not as solid as it had appeared at first. Thus the view that the prolongation of life is always good was eroded when it was suggested that there are times when it is not only efficient but humane to "let old Dad die," and extended consideration of the crushing burden of responsibility for selecting patients to receive dialysis concluded, as it had commenced, in a ring of uncertainty.

In a less excruciating way, the same kinds of conflict emerged as the group maneuvered to find the right place on the value scale for tender, loving care, which has been sinking in the rising tide of technology. Whether and how personal warmth and humaneness might be restored was debated at some length. Nobody was opposed to tender, loving care, exactly, but there were some who plainly felt it isn't really worth much worry, or much expense. No division was called for, but an observer guessed that if it had been, the hospital people would have come down on the side of professionalism and technology, and the social scientists would have come down in the milk of human kindness.

A vote on another value might have produced about the same result: The social scientists wanted more, or at least some, consumer participation in planning and conducting the health services, but the hospital administrators tended to think that papa knows best. In response to a sociologist who suggested that the consumer should have a share in decision making, a hospital administrator asked, "Why should we give the consumer a choice—because we value his freedom to choose, even if he makes a lousy choice?"

This was part of the reason, certainly, but there were other considerations, it developed. An economist noted that consumers are not altogether happy with the outcome of the health services and, through public bodies, are changing the way decisions are made. Others in the academic group said that consumers obviously aren't going to make medical decisions but the important thing is to give them a wider range of services to choose from than they have now. Since we clearly can't provide everything for everybody, the task is one of managing scarce resources, it was pointed out, and some of the decisions are thus beyond the competence of health professionals. A professor put the proposition bluntly: "This country is at a point where the provision of health care is a public utility, and the professionals are going to be ousted from making the decisions. Doctors in the future will be looked on as extraordinarily learned and talented plumbers."

Maybe doctors would like that, an administrator suggested, but he was joking. Even in the broad context of resource allocation, the medically oriented group doubted that consumers would make sensible choices: They place a high priority on getting well and a low priority on not getting sick; they make bad decisions and call on doctors to cope with the results; they want coronary care units everywhere but they won't stop smoking. We need values to measure cost benefits and to balance cost benefits to the individual and cost benefits to society on a price/utility scale, it was suggested. "If I were a dictator deciding on cost benefit to society, I'd abolish personal health services," said a sociologist, but this concept was quickly shot down: Benefit for both the individual and the society has to comprehend some degree of satisfaction and assign some value to quality—a circumstance that makes measurement fuzzy, if not impossible.

To some of the discussants the consideration of consumer participation centered in ghetto neighborhoods, where community engagement itself is a value that transcends others, including health, because the black communities, especially, simply won't accept services that are laid on for them by outsiders. The group heard how one inner-city neighborhood is organizing a communitywide nonprofit health agency that will contract with hospitals, physicians, group practices, welfare departments and other providers to furnish services. The community controls decisions about the services that are needed and decisions about staffing and budgeting, it was explained. The same community has taken the same approach to solution of its educational problems. "In this view the school is not an education system, but an instrument of public policy," said the urban affairs administrator, "and this is also true of the hospital. These patients increasingly approach the clinic declaring, 'This is what I want,' not, 'What have you got for me?' This is the only possible way to peace and progress for the ghetto. And we're finding that there's a lot of ability in there. There had to be, in order for these people to have survived."

This kind of community engagement may work in the ghetto and is needed in the ghetto because it is essential to the emerging process of self-identification of ghetto populations, it was generally agreed, but it wouldn't work, and isn't needed, elsewhere. In more affluent communities, consumer participation was seen as simply giving patients and families and well people a voice in the design and application of services. Patient and family expectations today are largely conditioned by physicians' values, a sociologist said, but they can easily be changed. Doctors and hospital administrators complain about irrational consumers, but what about irrational doctors who insist on hospitalization when it isn't needed? "Doctors could take the pressure off hospitals if they were organized to get the job done outside," the sociologist declared. "How are you going to control the doctor? Are you unwilling to take him on?"

The hospital people doubted that consumer organizations were an answer, or that hospital boards of trustees were generally representative of the consumer interest. Community advisory committees and patients' councils were suggested as possible mechanisms that might help make hospital care more palatable to consumers, but there was no great enthusiasm. "We have to be sure the quality of this institution doesn't deteriorate because of some outside interest," said an administrator whose mistrust of nonprofessional judgment was in plain view. "People would choose to have 25 bed hospitals, and we know they're no good," said another.

Possibly because they consistently tended to look at big rather than little causes and far rather than near effects, the economists took up a middle ground between the sociologists, who saw consumers as mostly ignored, and the hospital administrators, who saw them as just uninformed. Consumer interests are being recognized in the new public policy that describes health service as a right of all the people and in the new public policy that demands a place for consumers in health service planning, the economists pointed out. The trick now is to make right decisions about what services shall be included for all the people and what objectives shall guide planning—decisions enormously complicated by the ethic that says the quality of service must not vary according to the user's means and the law that says planning for public expense must comprehend the political process. "We must never say Joe Smith is alive because he could afford it and Bill Brown is dead because he couldn't," says the ethic, and, "You professionals are not going to run the whole show," says the law.

Medicare has provided the beginning, at least, of a description of the services that are considered a right or entitlement, but there was little agreement in this group, and there is little in the profession, or in the population, as to what the "basic bundle of services" should be. "Basic service is like the core curriculum," said an administrator. "It gets too big right away. The service floor is the floor of an elevator, and it's a tall building." There was agreement, however, that there must be a range of services, and that ways must be found for the consumer to "map his preferences into the outcome," as an economist put it, using one of his favorite phrases. "Hooking the consumer in on a mini-government scale may be the best way of finding an answer to the crucial question of balancing values and scarcities," he added, using another. Nobody had a better answer.

Whatever the process, the services that are wanted have to be planned, and unless the consumer is hooked into the planning input he isn't likely to get what he wants in the service outcome. Public Law 89-749 hooks the consumer into planning, all right, somebody observed, but this has not proved to be a cause for widespread rejoicing among either planners or professionals, who are contending with the states for control. Planning is too important to be left to planners, it was agreed. "I've seen how they use statistics, or what they think are statistics, and I don't want them making my plans," said an economist. Like hunters at dawn on opening day, everybody fired a round or two in the excitement, then settled down to figure out where the ducks were. "There are no standards or criteria for making right planning decisions," said a man who had been a member of the Secretary's Advisory Committee on Hospital Effectiveness. "The committee tried to set up some rules that would create the conditions for right political decisions."

That's the way to plan, an economist agreed. He called it structural planning, as opposed to prescriptive or "performance target" planning, in which "the consumer can easily be harnessed into a conspiracy against himself, pre-empting modalities and decreasing choices." What the consumer really wants is a way to get into the system, and out of it, with greater predictability, said the member of the Barr Committee. "But there are some real conflicts of interest in there," he warned. "Somebody's going to get hurt." He didn't say who, but it appeared that the best protection against injury in any case would be to make certain that all the right actors are in the play. One of the economists was skeptical. The system isn't doing such a bad job of responding to demand now, he suggested. "Why do you want to change it?" he asked. "You might make it worse."

The hospital people looked at one another as parents do over the head of an innocent child, silently choosing the one who will explain the facts of life. Then, "We are under bitter attack," the spokesman said quietly. "The system isn't going to stay the way it is. We are going to plan this way, with consumer interests represented, or we are going to have arbitrary pricing." Another spokesman added another point: "Let's not assume that decisions now are good," he said, putting a finger squarely on the reason doctors and hospitals don't want planning. "We have to compare two imperfect systems. Politics is forcing decisions based on demand. The art in planning is to give demand several inputs."

Up to now demand hasn't had much of any influence on planning, it was explained, because professional preferences have defined consumer preferences: I want what the doctor tells me I want. But the new public policy requires a new kind of planning, which was described as "a process of pitting people against one another"—providers, consumers, industry, government—on both the supply and demand sides, and "letting the system play." Letting the system play didn't sound like planning to the economists, but they had to put it down, finally, as another peculiarity of the health system—like the concept of a single standard of quality, which was described by a sociologist as "part of the professsional mythology, like lawyers assuming that all men are rational. It's something we have to contend with."

Here and elsewhere, the role of the hospital administrator, who spends a good part of his life in one way or another contending with professional mythology, was examined. The job is partly one of reconciling or accommodating conflicting forces and values within constraining budgets—a process one of the administrators described as applying "a thin layer of management on top of guilds of contending specialists." At the higher levels of skill, the administrator's job is also one of initiating pressures for improvement. The incentive for arousing trouble by pushing for change owes something to the desire to run a bigger show and something to the conviction that a bigger show is better for society, the administrators agreed, but they didn't say which came first. Either way, it isn't going to get any easier. The task of the administrator is increasingly one of external management, one of the wise men said, "—negotiating the existence of his institution against some very hard forces in a chancier world."

If the social sciences can contribute anything to the performance of that hard task—and the discussion here suggested that they can at least illuminate its complexities—the hospital administrator should invite them back again and again. He needs all the help he can get.

There Ought to Be
a Middle Ground

October 1975

Back home in California just before his resignation became effective, former Secretary of Health, Education and Welfare Caspar Weinberger made a speech criticizing the Congress for continuing to pile up social programs that promise to outrun the capability and willingness of the people to pay enough taxes to support them. It wasn't exactly an original thought. The difficulty has been examined by students and philosophers of government since the time of Plato's Republic, and its underlying cause was described by John Stuart Mill more than 100 years ago in his celebrated essay on representative government. "It is quite conclusive against any theory of government," he said, "that it assumes the numerical majority to do habitually what is never done, nor expected to be done, save in very exceptional cases, by any other depositaries of power—namely, to direct their conduct by their real ultimate interest, in opposition to their immediate and apparent interest."

Mill's faith in representative government was rooted in the basic assumptions that the representative assemblies would consist of superior intellects having the wisdom to resist, not encourage, the voters' interest in immediate and apparent beneficences for themselves, and that in any event the ministers would exercise restraint in disposing what the legislators authorized.

It hasn't worked out exactly that way. As Secretary Weinberger pointed out, the real ultimate interest of the people has taken second place right along to the immediate and apparent interest of the Congress in getting itself re-elected, and also, as the secretary didn't take occasion to emphasize, the ministers are often diverted from their devotion to the real ultimate interest of the people in order to pursue the chief minister's immediate and apparent interest in the same electoral objective, a pursuit that in Secretary Weinberger's time took some bizarre turns—not excluding the occasional tendency of the chief minister to consider that he was not chief minister but chief, period.

Foreseeing that ministers might not always remain aloof from the political hurly-burly, John Stuart Mill believed the chief minister should be appointed by the assembly, not elected by the voters. "Another important consideration is the great mischief of unintermitted electioneering," he said. "When the highest dignity in the state is to be conferred by popular election once in every four years, the whole intervening time is spent in what is virtually a canvass. Ministers, chiefs of party and their followers are all electioneerers, and every public question is discussed and decided with less reference to its merits than to its expected bearing on the election. If a system had been devised to make party spirit the ruling principle of action in all public affairs, it would have been difficult to contrive any means better adapted to the purpose." If he had anticipated that this was stating the case conservatively, the way things have turned out in the United States in the 1970s, Mr. Mill might readily have withdrawn his conclusion that, all things considered, representative government is still the best there is, and come out instead for kings and princes.

While Secretary Weinberger was not greatly beloved of those whose oxen were gored as he sought to apply the restraints he considered necessary to head off the slide into "egalitarian tyranny," as he described it, he must be credited with considering the real ultimate interest, as opposed to the immediate and apparent, at least as often as any ministers have done in our time, and a lot oftener than most of his, ah, classmates. Those drastic regulations for which he got sued as often as he was just blamed, he said, were made necessary by a Congress bent on "perpetuating a complex tangle of narrowly focused social programs." He didn't add that the administration of which he was a member had at first proposed to untangle the complex and broaden the focus by means of a welfare reform plan that was abandoned when interests that were more immediate and apparent obtruded. The plan was conceived and aborted before he got there, for one thing, and, for another, previous secretaries of HEW had reported trouble enough finding and counting the programs, so nobody ever really expected them to be untangled.

Mr. Weinberger's successor as secretary is being hailed on all sides as a brilliant young man who was making his mark as an educational administrator when the ink was scarcely dry on his diploma, though at 39 he could hardly be considered a prodigy in a society that is supposed to be youth oriented. Hospital and health professionals have been heard growling that he doesn't know an HMO from a sphygmomanometer, but that isn't necessarily bad, because it means he must let the knowledgeable and able professionals in the department tend to health affairs while he goes through the learning process that was explained by John Stuart Mill: "I have known public men, ministers, of more than ordinary natural capacity, who on their first introduction to a department of business new to them, have excited the mirth of their inferiors by the air with which they announced as a truth hitherto set at nought, and brought to light by themselves, which was probably the first thought of everybody who ever looked at the subject, given up as soon as he had got on to a second." Most ministers have to suffer this. Secretary Weinberger did, and, as a matter of fact, he may have added a new dimension to the experience by exciting some of the mirth at an early press conference. At any rate, it may comfort the health professionals to recall that the one HEW secretary who did know something about hospitals was so busy keeping up with the tergiversations of busing policy that he didn't have time for health matters. Anyway, by the time the present new secretary gets on to his second thought it is going to be 1976, and unintermitted electioneering will have set in again.

Dr. F. David Mathews is the third educator, and the second university president to become secretary of HEW. The other university president, is still around in government, appropriately engaged in affairs having to do with aging, and the other educator, possibly as a result of the HEW experience, has gone over to the other side and spent the last several years trying to reform the Congress—a task that must make HEW look easy. Others who have served terms at HEW have included a newspaper publisher, a businessman, two full-time and two part-time politicians, and a career civil servant whose effective dedication to what H.L. Mencken once called "organized lovey-dovey" may have been responsible for many of the programs Mr. Weinberger and friends were trying to untangle. In contrast to most of the others, the civil servant got things done. Whether that is good or bad, and whether a secretary succeeds or fails, depends not so much on what happens as it does on what is conceived to be the proper function of government. "A government which attempts to do everything is aptly compared to a schoolmaster who does all the pupils' tasks for them," said John Stuart Mill; "he may be very popular with the pupils, but he will teach them little. A government, on the other hand, which neither does anything itself that can possibly be done by anyone else, nor shows anyone else how to do anything, is like a school in which there is no schoolmaster, but only pupil teachers who have never themselves been taught." There ought to be a middle ground—if we could only leave off electioneering long enough to find it.

The Pressures Change;
The Conditions Remain

January 1979

This is the time of year when oracles multiply and flourish, producing always a predictable mixture of sanguinity and gloom. Thus the sales manager's bright vision of tomorrow's market is darkened by the certainty that bosses with long memories are taking note of his forecasts and will hold him responsible for any deficiencies. So also the politicians and public administrators, required by the custom that goes with the calendar to give their constituencies and jurisdictions a glimpse into the year ahead, must find some acceptable balance of promises dictated by elections and appointments yet to come and alarms called for by looming disappointments and disasters. As it does elsewhere in the society, the oracular pronouncement makes its seasonal appearance in the turbulent health care culture, where the oracles are busy performing their ritual tasks undeterred by the obvious fact that nobody knows what the hell is going to happen next week, let alone next year. Among the questions the health care oracles are expected to address again, as they have annually for the past decade and periodically for a generation or two before that, are the ones about national health insurance: Will we get it? What kind? How much? When?

Ever since the gods and goddesses of ancient Greece looked for guidance from the priestess Pythia in the temple at Delphi, oracles have commonly begun their divinations about the future by reviewing the past, and there seems no good reason for an ink-stained amateur prophet to depart from the practice now. Looking at the long sweep of the past, even a part-time oracle can easily see that interest in national health insurance has been rising and receding for 50 or 60 years, peaking briefly after World War I, when a few public health leaders became fascinated with the development of sickness insurance in Europe; and again in the early 1930s when health insurance for all Americans was recommended by the Committee on the Costs of Medical Care, producing shudders of horror in hospital board rooms; and again in the late 1940s when Social Security Administrator Oscar Ewing and Senator Robert Wagner of New York and the United Auto Workers, among others, came close; and again in the Great Society push of the 1960s, when we got what we've got. All the peaks and valleys of interest have been responses to varying pressures of economics and politics that only rarely have risen to the level of real public debate, as opposed to the semipublic debate that involves only politicians, bureaucrats, and special interest groups and might be described as foam without beer. The last time there was beer we got Medicare and Medicaid, whose existence suggests that for the past 10 years the oracles have been addressing the wrong questions. We already have national health insurance, and the right question now is whether or not we shall have more.

As recently as a half dozen years ago, nearly everybody seemed to have agreed that we should have. A Republican president had proposed a Family Health Insurance Plan to go along with his Family Assistance Plan for welfare reform, and as it was described later by Daniel P. Moynihan, the White House welfare specialist at the time who later became a United States Senator, "FHIP was to Medicaid as FAP was to Aid to Families with Dependent Children." An effort to broaden the coverage and iron out the inequities of Medicaid, FHIP would have covered five or six million families at premiums ranging from zero, for families with incomes up to $1,600, to $500 for those at $5,600, the upper limit of eligibility for public assistance then. FHIP and FAP were stillborn, as it turned out; liberals opposed the plans because they were too stingy, according to Moynihan, and the administration got involved with wage and price controls and other preoccupations. So FHIP evaporated, but it was an important milestone nevertheless; for the first time, a conservative Republican administration had acknowledged the need for something more than a liberal Democratic Congress had provided. It wasn't clear then, and isn't clear yet, whether the need seen by conservatives has been one for medical assistance for deprived populations or popular assistance for deprived politicians; either way, the issue gained respectability and has never again dropped completely out of sight. The ebb and flow of interest continues, but the tempo is livelier. The

AMA, AHA, insurance companies, Blue Cross and Blue Shield, labor, and even groups like the U.S. Chamber of Commerce are all in there now, year after year, testifying in empty hearing rooms and arguing what kind and how much. Unfortunately for the millions who are caught in the cracks between public and private programs, there isn't the faintest glimmer of agreement on just what it is that is needed or what the nation will hold still to pay for, and it will take some consensus on both points to get another entitlement.

The one thing the Congress might be persuaded to consider is a proposal that would mandate some form of catastrophic expense coverage that wouldn't cost too much and wouldn't help too much but would permit the maximum of breastbeating on television about those exorbitant doctors' and hospital bills. And if this were to be combined with a minimum pass at pouring a little more federal wine in state Medicaid bottles, it could be, and would be called national health insurance, and its sponsors and supporters could be seen as, or at least pose as, heroes. The only trouble with this is that once the Congress passed an entitlement it could call national health insurance, it would be inclined to put the issue back on the shelf, and the hapless people who are stuck in the cracks would probably be there for another 10 years.

Who are they?

Principally, they are the poor and the near poor whose incomes are over Medicaid eligibility limits in states where the limits are unrealistically low, and the poor and near poor in states where eligibility and benefits have been cut back because the states are running out of money. Also stuck in the cracks are all but the comfortably well off among the nation's aged—a group that is growing at the rate of 1,500 or more a day. Medicare pays only an estimated 40 per cent of their total medical expenses, and the percentage is going down as costs rise and deductibles are increased. For the aged on limited fixed incomes, and that includes most of them, inflation is not just a nagging worry but a cruel hardship. Besides the poor and the old, there are still uncounted millions in the work force whose families are uninsured or inadequately protected. As hospital financial managers know better than most others, some of those hundreds of insurance companies writing hospital and medical expense policies are shell games run by carnival hucksters in pinstripes.

Right now it looks as though the pressures to save money and hold down taxes will remain stronger than the pressures to get the poor and the old and the underinsured out of the cracks. But sooner or later the pressures will be reversed, not just because the politicians will come to a different estimate of what will make them look good back home, but chiefly because between elections the majority of them are decent men and women who want to do the right thing, and the right thing in the concept most of us believe in is to make it as certain as we can that those who are struck down by misfortune are given the opportunity to stand again. The combination of illness and poverty is the worst of misfortunes, certainly, and if we have to accept the added burden of some welfare cheats and their medical equivalents in order to redress the misfortunes of the sick poor and the aged, ultimately we shall.

Contemplating Medicare cost reports, Medicaid cutbacks, late payments, retroactive denials, and the frustrating ambiguities of bureacratic management, hospital people wince at the thought that more national health insurance would inevitably bring larger segments of the population into what most of them see as mismanaged systems. When a federal official at a recent hospital meeting mentioned Medicare as a government department that works well, everybody laughed—but with overtones of hysteria. But it does work, and the fact that Medicare for all its infirmities works so much better than Medicaid does should offer some hope that a FHIP might be better, not worse, than what we've got. It is at least possible that when it comes, more national health insurance may be an extension of the private more than of the public system, an end devoutly to be wished and lobbied for, not because private insurers are brighter and better than bureaucrats, which may be true or untrue in any given case, but because they have different jobs, as a professor in the Graduate School of Business Administration at New York University once explanied. "Bureaucratic management is management bound to comply with detailed rules and regulations fixed by the authority of a superior body," Professor Ludwig von Mises wrote. "In public administration there is no market price for achievement. This makes it indispensable to operate public offices according to principles entirely different from those applied under the profit motive. The citizen compares the operation of the bureau with the working of the profit system, which is more familiar to him. Then he discovers that bureaucratic management is wasteful, inefficient, slow, and rolled up in red tape. He simply cannot understand how reasonable people allow such a mischievous system to endure. Such criticisms are not sensible. They misconstrue the features peculiar to public administration. If one goes to their roots, one often learns that they are not simply the result of culpable negligence or lack of competence. They sometimes turn out to be the result of special political or institutional conditions, or of an attempt to come to an arrangement with a problem for which a more satisfactory solution could not be found. A detailed scrutiny of all the difficulties involved may convince an honest investigator that, given the general state of political forces, he himself would not have known how to deal with the matter in a less objectionable way."[1]

It is possible to agree with Professor von Mises, at least in part, without giving up the conviction that there has to be a less objectionable way to run a national health insurance system, and that one such way would be to insist on a larger share of responsibility for private insurers.

However, the private insurance system as a government contractor is not the same thing as the private insurance system as a private contractor, and even if it were, that wouldn't resolve what may be the underlying disjunction of the public financing system we've got now, and the private insurance system we've got now, and any extension we may get of either one. The disjunction is that we are using and paying a medical care system for a multitude of purposes that are only faintly related to medical care and some that aren't related at all. It has been suggested that this all began when Medicare came along and we started talking about "health care" instead of "medical care" and "hospital care," in order to accommodate the needs of the elderly, who were obviously going to require many services that have more to do with social support than with medical care. Unquestionably, the practice of using the medical care system as a social support system was expanded and accelerated by Medicare, which is supporting thousands of aged patients in hospitals and nursing homes not because they are sick but because they have no place else to go.

But the practice began long before Medicare. In fact, comfort, advice, counseling, guidance, home services—elements of care that are more social than medical—were a large part of what the general practitioner of our grandfathers' time offered his patients, and their roots go deep into the origins of medicine in religious institutions that were havens for the homeless sick. The reemergence of these elements now in the concept of "health care" presents staggering burdens, partly because medical care *per se* has become so specialized, so complex, so technological, so intellectually and scientifically demanding, but mostly because the need for comfort and counseling and support today involves not just the sick but virtually the entire population. An example in everyday practice is the use of ataractic drugs, which took off from their base in psychiatry, where there was never any question about their usefulness in helping the mentally ill and disabled, and have come to be used by all kinds of physicians for all kinds of purposes, many of which have nothing to do with illness. Harassed by the pressures and stresses of a machine-ridden industrial society, the population looks increasingly to medicine for answers medicine hasn't got, and more people see more doctors more times for more reasons than our present financing systems, geared to pay for medical care *qua* medical care, can possibly comprehend. "The goals of the health care system traditionally emphasized reduction of death and disability, and also relief of distress," said Dr. Gerald Klerman, professor of psychiatry at Harvard Medical School and former administrator of HEW's Alcohol, Drug Abuse and Mental Health Administration. "It is the extension of the definition of distress that leads to the policy dilemma. In the past, distress involved bodily pain, as in broken limbs and abdominal catastrophes. However, in the current era the definition of distress has been broadened to include emotional and psychic complaints including anxiety, tension, insomnia, and personal and social misfortunes. The health care system is being called upon not only to reduce mortality and disability but also to relieve distressing symptoms and increasingly to enhance our capacities for performance and happiness."[2]

Dr. Klerman and others believe that the definition of illness must be determined by public policy, and the "medical necessity" provisions in Medicare and insurance are an effort to cut down the extravagant costs of social malaise masquerading as illness. But if people keep on wanting to go to doctors and hospitals to have their anxieties treated and their happiness enhanced, public policy pronouncements probably aren't going to stop them, and neither are medical necessity rules and PSROs. Physicians who don't like patients who aren't really sick usually can find ways to discourage them, but these patients eventually find doctors willing to help, at least by listening—and who can say that isn't as useful and noble a calling as excising a diseased appendix? Critics argue that listening and handholding and head-patting can be done by nurses and clergy and maybe Boy Scouts, but the patients don't want nurses or clergy or Boy Scouts.They want doctors, preferably in white coats.

Will it ever be possible to develop a health care system in which needs like this can be managed, and still provide for those who have been left out? Nobody knows. But it is certain that the effort to do both will continue, with more, and more stringent, medical necessity rules, and more deductibles, and more incentives and alternatives, aimed at limiting social uses of medical resources, and with more pressures, including the pressure to do the right thing, aimed at getting the outcasts inside the system. As it has in the past, the struggle will go on a step at a time, with some sidesteps and backsteps, in response to varying economic and political tensions, not declarations of policy. And whether it succeeds or not may depend as much as anything on the effectiveness of the new surge of interest in health education of the public. Especially, it may depend on convincing physicians that the survival of their profession the way they want it may be determined by their willingness to join the effort to get people who aren't really sick to stay home. Those without homes can't be wholly the responsibility of doctors and hospitals. That's what public policy is for.

[1]von Mises, L., Bureaucratic Management, in de Huszar, George B., ed., Fundamentals of Voluntary Health Care, Caldwell, ID: Caxton Printers, Ltd., 1962.

[2]Klerman, G.L., Mental Health: Recommendations for Public Policy. Presented at the Conference on Future Directions in Health Care, sponsored by the Institute of Medicine, the Rockefeller Foundation, the Blue Cross Association, and the Health Policy Program, University of CA at San Francisco, New York, February 15, 1977.

Services for Whom?
What for?

November 1975

It was a dozen or so years ago when the Citizens Commission on Graduate Medical Education headed by John Millis, Ph.D., turned the spotlight on primary care and started all the arguments about how the primary physician should be trained, and for what. The spotlight is still on, and so are the arguments. The Millis report chose, if it did not invent, the term primary physician, in preference to family physician, to emphasize its concept of the role as first contact and prime resource, desirably but not necessarily or invariably family counselor. Sometimes there isn't any family. As it turned out, however, the action went the other way. There are now more than 200 family practice training programs in community hospitals and university medical centers and new ones are still being organized. Family doctor is an honorable, though not exactly glamorous, title, but by a precise inversion of language that may be peculiar to medicine, everybody understands that primary means second-rate. Who wants it? The best and the brightest still swarm the overcrowded surgical specialties and the strata of internal medicine, like molecular biology, at the furthest remove from primary care. This in spite of the fact that emphasis on training for primary care has been a major goal of the Association of American Medical Colleges for the past several years, and everybody from the assistant dean for undergraduate studies to the President of the United States has been crying the need for somebody to look at the sore throats and listen to the anxieties, not just take something out and send it to the laboratory.

For all the uproar, however, sore throats and anxieties remain at the fringes of medical interest, whose core is the removable or repairable organ or part. So now we are training a gallimaufry of nurses, corpsmen, technicians, aides, assistants and associates to cope with the people's problems so physicians will have time enough to read the oscillographs and lab reports and order the next round of tests. This isn't going to work either, for reasons that were made clear by a hospital patient who was visited by one of Sociologist Hans Mauksch's investigators. "What kind of day are you having?" the researcher asked. "I've had a wonderful day," the patient beamed. "I got to talk to my doctor!" Assistants can do everything but satisfy the patients.

The reasons nothing much has changed in the past decade are complex and probably not fully understood by anybody, but it seems likely that if it were the professional educators who decided what kind of medicine the society should have, by this time we'd have primary physicians coming out of our ears. But it isn't the professionals who tell the society, it's the society that tells the professionals, and plainly the society is still enchanted by the miracles of the operating rooms and intensive care areas and laboratories. So miracle makers are what the society has been getting and will continue to get until the market for miracles cools off and the market for medical counseling begins to pick up.

There are some signs that this may happen. Disenchantment with miracles has already set in, not for any lack of miracle makers but partly because miracles were oversold, mostly on television, to the point where anything short of loaves and fishes was seen as malpractice, and partly because it's hard to have a trusting relationship with a miracle maker, let alone a machine, and partly because there were so many miracle makers around producing miracles and near miracles that weren't always needed that the whole business got awfully expensive. Another sign has been the somewhat diminished traffic at the front door of the hospital and the traffic jams at the back door, where miracles are not unknown but the staple is a pat on the head and a band-aid. Still another sign is the burgeoning of departments of community medicine, and social medicine, and family practice, and health education, and the rising interest of medical schools and teaching hospitals in affiliations with community hospitals in response to the awakening realization that the reason young physicians whose entire clinical experience has been in coronary care units don't want to treat bee-stings and sprains is not just that they aren't interested but that they don't know how. The surgical resident on outpatient duty who treats a runny nose with a cold shoulder may be not so much arrogant or impatient as he is afraid of looking foolish. The thing that is in short supply around a lot of hospitals today is not money or manpower, but comfort. It isn't hard to understand why. Asked about the trend toward training more primary care physicians, a professor of medicine at one of the nation's great teaching institutions said it wasn't anything more than "the latest fad in medical education." With teachers like that, who's looking for high marks in tender loving care?

There is a school of revolutionary thought that favors oppression of the masses on the ground that the worse things get, the sooner the people will rise, and there are medical radicals who would like to see hospitals get more expensive and impersonal and thus hasten the overthrow of the system. In both medicine and politics, the motives of reformers who want to keep the system intact but improve its performance to curb dissatisfactions that could result in overthrow are frequently misunderstood, with the result that reformers are seen by some as enemies instead of friends. Thus the call for a rein on specialization and technology, and emphasis instead on comfort and care, may be considered either a sin against the culture or essential to its survival, but whatever it is, it is growing in volume and intensity, reflecting the increasing disposition of the society to expect more from doctors and hospitals, and not get it.

Inevitably, many of the most urgent calls for reform are coming from critics outside the profession, as in books like Victor Fuchs' "Who Shall Live?" Ivan Illich's "Medical Nemesis," and Rick Carlson's "End of Medicine." But it may be significant that the signals are also rising within the medical establishment. One such comes from Victor W. Sidel, M.D., chairman of the department of social medicine at the Montefiore Hospital and Medical Center and Albert Einstein College of Medicine in New York, who suggested in a recent paper that determinations of quality in medical care necessarily must be made by measurements of performance against some model or goal, and that up to now the professional goals have emphasized the technical aspects of care at the expense of the emotional, social and economic factors in illness and without regard for such basic questions as: "For whom are services to be provided? To what end are they given? A more specific, and in my view more important, way of putting the questions is: Are the services directed toward those who already have much, or toward those who have relatively little? Are they directed toward redressing the balance or do they, in effect if not in conscious design, widen the gap between those who have and those who have not?"[1] The only way to get considerations like these into measurements of healthcare quality, according to Dr. Sidel, is to get nonprofessionals involved in making the measurements, which are certain to reflect professional views and values so long as they are the sole responsibility of professionals.

Dr. Sidel's prescription is not likely to be cheered unrestrainedly by many physicians, nor by anybody else who has had anything to do with the current efforts to define and measure quality, including a lot of hospital administrators and trustees who are coping nervously with their newly recognized need to master this arcane art. But it can be seen nevertheless as facing in the direction in which events are moving, toward the time when patients will be people, and primary physicians will be primary, and the focus of healthcare will be health. It won't be next week.

[1]Sidel, Victor W., M.D., Quality for Whom? Effects of Professional Responsibility for Quality of Health Care on Equity, presented at the 1975 annual health conference of the New York Academy of Medicine, "The Professional Responsibility for Quality of Health Care," April 24-25, 1975.

All the Worse for the Fishes

The point about overproduction and overemphasis on technology was being made repeatedly, and among many who were writing books about it were the reformers whose prescriptions for the health care system are reviewed here: Ivan Illich: Abolish It. Rick Carlson: Shrink It. Victor Fuchs: Change It.

June 1975

The institutionalized aged are the most seriously damaged victims of industrialized society—worse off even than the poor in backward countries, who have learned to survive by making do on their own. The elderly in U.S. hospitals and nursing homes, in contrast, have been robbed of their ability to cope with their illnesses and their environments by the medical establishment, which has been industrialized along with everything else in the society. These and other equally cheerless views of health care today have been fashioned into a chilling assessment of doom by Ivan Illich, the priest-philosopher-educator whose Center for Intercultural Documentation is a social issues think tank with headquarters at Cuernavaca, Mexico, and tentacles reaching into three continents. Mr. Illich declares that the elderly in the United States are an extreme example of suffering promoted by high cost deprivation. "Having learned to consider old age akin to disease," he says, "they develop unlimited economic needs paying for interminable therapies which are usually ineffective, frequently demeaning and painful, and which most often require recovery in a special milieu." These are among the less censorious judgments in "Medical Nemesis—The Expropriation of Health," a book by Mr. Illich. "The book has already raised much controversy in the press and in medical papers in France and England," said a review by a professor of psychology at London University. "It is an effective polemical expression of the diffuse dissatisfaction with medicine which has been gathering force for the last decade or so."

This is a nice way of saying that Mr. Illich thinks medicine does more harm than good. This is, in fact, the basic postulate of "Medical Nemesis," and its impact on the medical establishment may be compared to what happened 150 years ago when Lobachevsky constructed a whole new world of mathematical thought on the assumption that parallel lines may converge. "It can hardly be imagined how shocking the denial of one of Euclid's assumptions must have seemed at the time," a mathematics scholar wrote recently, possibly anticipating what medical historians may one day say about Mr. Illich, who describes medical nemesis as "the expropriation of man's coping ability and his maintenance at the service of the industrial system." Contemporary medicine, he explains, suffers from one distinguishing delusion: "It assumes that all the ills of everyone ought to be treated, whatever the predictable outcome. Unfortunately, this therapeutic mania is infectious and has crippled the traditional art of sick care . . . When the dependence on the professional management of pain, sickness and death grows beyond a certain threshold, the healing power in sickness, patience in suffering, and fortitude in the face of death must decline. These three regressions are symptoms of third-level iatrogenesis; their combined outcome is medical nemesis." The other two levels of iatrogenesis are the undesirable side effects of approved, mistaken, callous or contraindicated contacts with the medical system, such as the use of harmful drugs for minor ailments, which Mr. Illich has classified as clinical iatrogenesis, and the encouragement of sickness, as in institutionalization, or breeding demands for the patient's role, which he labels social iatrogenesis.

Mr. Illich's strictures about treatments that are laid on without regard for outcome are not just talk. In this and other sections, the book is liberally documented with references to the medical and social literature of the United States, Canada, Great Britain, France, Germany and Latin America. Here, for example, he refers to studies showing doubtful results of high technology: treatment of myocardial infarction, the futility of the tonsillectomies still performed on a substantial fraction of the healthy children in the population; the socialization of diagnosis through automated multiphasic screening, which not only "has no impact on life expectancy" but "helps to transfer people who feel healthy into anxious patients," and, especially, indiscriminate medication. "Public fascination with medical breakthroughs, high technology care, and death under medical control is a symptom of the intense medicalization of our culture," Mr. Illich says in a vintage paragraph. "It can best be understood as a deep-seated need for miracle cures. The gaudy care is financed, like the liturgies of old, by taxes, gifts and sacrifices. White coats, antiseptic environments, cancer research, ambulances and insurance serve magical and symbolic functions influencing health." Mr. Illich denies that the unneeded shot of penicillin may still have a useful placebo effect. "As drugs become more effective, their symbolic side effects have become overwhelmingly health-denying," he insists. "Instead of mobilizing the patient's self-healing powers, modern medical magic turns the patient into a limp and mystified onlooker upon whom procedures are performed."

Of course, not all these jaundiced judgments of medical performance are newly minted by Mr. Illich. As long ago as the 1850s Cardinal Newman was discoursing about "the physician who has so simply fixed his intellect on his own science as to have forgotten the existence of any other" and who thus considered himself "free to insist upon rules which are quite insufferable to any religious mind and antagonistic to faith and morals." Nor have animadversions on medicine been restricted to the religious: In one of his celebrated essays on medicine, Oliver Wendell Holmes suggested that with the exception of a few natural herbs the whole *materia medica* could be sunk to the bottom of the sea and "it would be all the better for mankind, and all the worse for the fishes." For the most part, however, the latter day critics of medicine, inside and outside the profession, have contended only that prescribed treatments are often useless. It is at the core of Mr. Illich's recusancy that such treatment is positively damaging to the patient because it dehumanizes by robbing him of the will and ability to cope for himself and depriving him of what Mr. Illich considers to be the natural human experiences of pain and suffering. Mr. Illich's rationale for this reversal of medical values leans heavily on our cultural and religious heritage and at times disappears into mysticism, emerging again to remind us that pain is often a useful signal having special meaning for physicians as well as patients.

"Pain loses its referential character if it is dulled and generates a meaningless, questionless, residual horror," he declares. "The new experience that has replaced dignified suffering is artificially prolonged, opaque, depersonalized maintenance. Increasingly, painkilling turns people into feelingless spectators of their own decaying selves." So also with death, which has been expropriated and industrialized, along with illness, "as society, acting through the medical system, decides when and after what indignities we shall die." The medicalization of society has brought the epoch of natural death to an end, Mr. Illich believes. "Mechanical death has conquered and destroyed all other deaths."

These and other Illich meditations do not go down easily among the purveyors of modern medicine, any more than his views on education evoked cheering in the quadrangles when "Deschooling Society" was published a few years ago. In a review of "Medical Nemesis," for example, Prof. D.W. Harding complained that Mr. Illich deprives medicine of the credit for its obvious advances, as in the declining mortality from infectious disease. "When Illich concludes that the professional practice of physicians cannot be given credit for these advances in health he is grotesquely narrowing the range of medical work and influence," says Prof. Harding, who is willing to acknowledge nevertheless that Mr. Illich is "raising issues responsible doctors are not inclined to brush aside." Others are less charitable, as when an Australian physician argued in the *British Medical Journal* that whereas neither high cost technological medicine nor the simplistic medicine that Mr. Illich believes in will meet all the needs of large populations, "decisions about the mixture of the two must still remain largely with the doctors, and statements about medicine made by amateurs such as Illich demonstrate only how little they understand. They do not understand what medicine is, nor what it can achieve, nor what its claims are. The medical profession is at least as self critical as any other body of people, and probably more so than most. Nothing said by Illich has not already been said by some doctor."

It is undeniably true that the medical profession has been self-critical, probably since the time of Hippocrates and probably more so than any others. But it can't be true that doctors have already said everything Mr. Illich has set down in "Nemesis," where he concluded that "the true miracle of modern medicine is diabolical. It consists of making not only individuals but whole populations survive on inhumanly low levels of personal health. By refusing medicine each one can question the social base of industrial society at that point at which it is most intimately entrenched." Any doctor who understands what that means couldn't say it. Move over, Marx.

Less Medicine Than
We Think

December 1975

Exercise, nutrition, diet, air, water, waste, light, sound, housing, recreation, work, stress, congestion, attitude, motivation and medical care are all known to be related to health, though little is known about the relative importance of their influence on health. Yet nearly all the funds available for health are poured into medical care, with practically none for all the other factors—not even to find out how, and how much, they do affect health. This doesn't make any sense, as some leaders of thought in medicine and the related biological and social sciences are beginning to point out, and it may help explain what a professor of psychology at London University referred to recently as "the diffuse dissatisfaction with medicine which has been gathering forces for the last decade or so." Some critics have stated the proposition in less conservative terms. One of these is Rick J. Carlson, whose book "The End of Medicine" (New York: John Wiley & Sons, 1975) argues that the entire medical enterprise has less impact on health than social and environmental factors have, and a new approach is required that will involve abandoning, or dismembering, the existing medical care system and designing a new, leaner system based on a new concept of health.

In this concept, health is not simply the absence of disease or impairment, as is commonly considered to be the case, nor is it a state or condition that achieves and maintains the ability to cope or function; it is rather a continuing process of adaption and interaction with environmental, social and personal forces. Thus, Mr. Carlson: "The passing view, derived largely from a mechanistic world view, assumes that human beings and nature are competitors and hence that human survival is dependent on control and manipulation of nature. This is also the premise of modern medicine.... To think of health as a process of man-environment interaction does not entail dividing the sick and the well into separate camps. Health and disease are not separate states or qualities. We do not move from one state to another as if changing clothes. Rather, health and disease are part of a process or continuum, mutually interdependent aspects of a situation." In this view, as Mr. Carlson has pointed out, the sick can be healthy. It is not an easy concept to grasp, especially for physicians, whose traditional mode of thought dates back to Hippocrates' discourse *On Ancient Medicine*: "Let us inquire then what is admitted to be Medicine; namely, that which was invented for the sake of the sick, which possesses a name and practitioners, whether it also seeks to accomplish the same objects, and whence it derived its origin."

Given his perspective of health, it is not hard to understand Mr. Carlson's disenchantment with a medical care system that keeps pouring out more and more money and manpower and machines and getting back less and less improvement in the health status of the population. But that isn't all. Like Ivan Illich, whose "Medical Nemesis" is a briefer and fiercer polemic of the same order of argument, Mr. Carlson considers that one of the effects of the swelling medical system has been the "medicalization" of personal and social problems such as aging, alcoholism, drug addiction, and pregnancy, with the result that patients have lost confidence in their ability to take care of themselves. Medicine shouldn't be criticized for seeking to treat such problems if it has the tools to help, he acknowledges, but it doesn't have, except rarely. Yet "as medicine encroaches on more of human life, it further incapacitates its major ally—the patient—for assuming responsibility for health." Medicine's disease-oriented approach to health also overlooks what Mr. Carlson calls "a blizzard of phenomena about the human being, because it does not fit medicine's paradigm of healing."

Inevitably, the disease-oriented approach takes us through the door to the hospital, which Mr. Carlson describes as one of the unhealthiest places around, whose purpose is to classify, confine and immobilize. "Admission is contingent on appropriate classification of a disease condition," says Mr. Carlson, listing as evil what the Social Security Administration would consider good. "The patient is then confined in quarters that are much the same everywhere. This is because to the physician the human being is simply a machine with interchangeable parts.

A given disease can be treated identically in Peoria or in Phoenix; it is the disease that is being treated, not the person. Today's medicine has succeeded where the medicines of the past have failed: It has succeeded in equating medical care with health. But the borders of the paradigm are blurring. It is becoming increasingly clear that health is not the same as medicine. The wrong questions have deservedly received the wrong answers. A new paradigm for health is slowly emerging. The medicine of today pits man against a hostile world. But it is in the relationship between human beings and their environment that the key to health lies. Health then is not just the well-oiled functioning of the body; it is achieved through the strategic collaboration of human beings with their world, expressed through a series of relationships. The physician can help, but the individual must be responsible for those relationships."

The relationships Mr. Carlson has in mind come in all varieties—personal, natural, spiritual. In fact, he is fascinated by—not to say hooked on—the supernatural, and he has a lot to say about astrology, extrasensory perception, psychokinesis and other paranormal phenomena, not excluding Carlos Castaneda's "Don Juan" and even Philippine psychic surgery, of which he observes, in a passage that is not unreasonable but unlikely to amass affirmative votes in the doctor's lounge, "The skeptic suggests that the case is one of patent fraud. This is a reasonable question, but there is a far more pertinent one: What difference does it make to the patient? The principal objection of modern medicine to unconventional healing is that it is fraudulent, that it fails to utilize accepted tools and techniques, in short that it is unscientific. The result is that the battle between modern medicine and other therapies is joined on the wrong question. One of the reasons that the question is not being asked is that the answer is potentially embarrassing. This is not to say that fraud is widespread in today's medicine, but rather to say that the question of fraud is irrelevant if a healthy outcome to the patient is the concern."

As a health services research attorney for InterStudy, the Minneapolis medical care think tank, and, later, a consultant to the Institute of Medicine, National Academy of Sciences, and adjunct assistant professor of medicine at Boston University school of medicine, Mr. Carlson has worked around the fringes of the medical profession long enough to understand that the argument that medicine has come to a point where there is no place to go but back is certain to encounter fierce opposition, and he has been at pains to anticipate and deflect attack, including the charge that boils down to the familiar, "you can't change human nature." His answer: It isn't easy, but it isn't impossible. The public demand for more and more medicine as it is known today frustrates the new approach, he admits. "I have not argued that the revolution can be accomplished in six days with a day of rest," he counters. "It will take a long time, and medicine will oppose the changes I propose. Others will argue that I have overstated the case. Perhaps I have. Medicine can and does cure. All I have said is that it cures far less than is generally understood, and that its modalities of treatment, whether effective or not, can cause more ill health than is cured. All that I have argued, peeled to its core, is that the size, scope and cost of medicine be reduced and calibrated with its relative influence on the ultimate goal—healthy individuals and a healthy population."

How do we get there from here? In the main, what Mr. Carlson offers is a compass, not a road map: less professionalism, fewer restrictions on healing, diminished use of hospitals and technology for other than acute care; more health education, more prevention, more research in behavior, greater use and choice of healing and helping personnel; investigation and push on social and environmental barriers to health. Mr. Carlson sums it up in a sentence: "We are on a high technology-low humanism trajectory in health, but a shift is possible—a shift to a medicine with a low technology and high humanism."

Put that simply, it doesn't sound impossible, but what we are likely to get instead, before the imbalance seen by Messrs. Carlson, Illich and others can be redressed, is enactment by the Congress of a comprehensive entitlement to medical care that will open the gates a little wider, increase the traffic on the familiar paths, and make any change in direction harder to accomplish. The reason it will happen this way was once made clear by the British economist Harold Lasswell. "All political decisions," he said, "are determinations of who gets what."

Other Functions, Other Flags

October 1974

Put together PSRO, HMO, PAS, QAP, PEP, HUR, PUR, HASP, MARP, CHAMP and any other monitoring or data system that may be strangling in its own printouts, and you still haven't got as effective a method of controlling utilization as one simple, tested measure would provide: Take away beds till it hurts. When Milton Roemer, Mike Anderson, Doug Colman, and a few others were pointing this out 20 years ago, give or take, the reaction was a combination of disbelief and disdain, as might happen if a physician were to diagnose warts and recommend amputation. "Beds that are built will be occupied," said Dr. Roemer, and everybody thought, "Why is that bad?" "The only effective utilization committees are in areas with bed shortages," said Mr. Anderson, and everybody around thought he was joking.

But when lesser measures prove ineffective and warts multiply and show signs of malignancy, amputation has to be taken seriously, or at least more seriously. In this case, the new consultant is Victor R. Fuchs, a health economist with a chestful of merit badges, a drawerful of name foundation grants, and the rare economist's ability to make a radical proposal appear to be the only course of action anybody in his right mind could consider. In a book published last year [1] but not widely acclaimed at first outside the tight little island of health economists and intellectuals, Mr. Fuchs identified excessive hospital capacity as the major cause of health care costs that have got out of hand and proposed a five-year moratorium on hospital expansion as the treatment of choice.

Mr. Fuchs doesn't say in so many words that PSRO, PAS, QAP and company won't work. In fact, he doesn't even mention them. The only one of the new constructs that is given any house room here at all is HMO, which is examined under the microscope and given a passing grade but finds its way only indirectly into the prescriptive regimen that is the compulsory coda of economists' compositions: "Capitation payment that covers hospitalization, medical care, and drugs has proven in practice to be convenient for the patient and easy to administer," this says. "Most important of all, it leads to significant reductions in cost without jeopardizing health."

A central theme of the Fuchs composition is that physicians make all the important decisions, including hospital decisions. "From the point of view of the hospital administrator, running a hospital is like trying to drive a car when the passengers have control of the wheel and the accelerator," he says. "The most the administrator can do is occasionally jam on the brakes." The analogue would hold up better, actually, if the physicians were seen controlling the brakes, as when they walked out of hospitals recently in San Francisco, New York, and elsewhere, while the harassed administrator is at the wheel, trying to steer around the obstacles. But the point nevertheless is an important one that isn't always fully understood; regulations that seek to control physicians by penalizing hospitals, as so many have done, are an unhappy example of how this basic relationship may be misread by those who should know better.

As heavy thinkers sometimes do when exploring new territory, to the delight or dismay of those already familiar with the coastline, Mr. Fuchs occasionally plants a flag of discovery on land that has been under cultivation for years. This is the case, for example, when he examines the complex interconnections of hospital size, function and efficiency and concludes, as if *de novo*, that "all the hospitals in a given area should be functionally integrated so that there can be an easy flow of patients and physicians from one facility to another depending upon medical requirements and available space"—an idea that has been around at least since the report of the Committee on the Costs of Medical Care in the 1930s and rediscovered repeatedly since that time by every committee, commission, bureau or agency that has looked at the subject for more than a few minutes. To his credit, Mr. Fuchs understands the reason it hasn't happened: "The notion of merging with a better-managed hospital, or of going out of business altogether, is not easily accepted by those with a large emotional stake in a particular hospital."

Another flag planted by Mr. Fuchs a few years ago in a

journal article and referred to here is the use of third-party reimbursement, and especially prospective reimbursement, for control of utilization and cost. "There is no reason why the third-party reimburser could not raise or lower the adjustment factor for particular services that it wished to encourage or discourage," he points out, explaining how the system would work. When Mr. Fuchs first proposed it in 1969, the idea was not as shopworn as it is today, but Blue Cross plans, among others, had already been tinkering with it for years and found out why it doesn't work: Hospitals don't care that much about saving money. As Mr. Fuchs explains it here, " Shrouded in the mantle of 'nonprofit' and convinced of the worthiness of all their endeavors, hospital administrations have been primarily concerned with justifying high costs rather than considering whether the resources siphoned into the hospital field might not be better used in other directions, including other dimensions of healthcare. Moreover, even when administrators attempt to take a broader view, their freedom to act is sharply limited by the hospital's physicians on the one hand and the board of trustees on the other."

Here as elsewhere, Mr. Fuchs has examined all the possible exits and come back to the same narrow window: The only escape from high costs is through physician behavior. Thus capitation payments, use of physicians' assistants, and control of physician supply by restraints on residencies are all parts of his prescribed economic regimen, along with universal health insurance and, finally, the bed moratorium, which is seen not just as an instrument of utilization control but also as a needed brake on what Mr. Fuchs describes as the monotechnic view of physicians. Trained in the application of a particular technology, the person with this view fails to recognize the claims of competing wants or the divergence of his priorities from those of other people, so his advice is likely to be a poor guide to social policy, Mr. Fuchs explains. Thus "a five-year moratorium on new bed capacity would be salutary and would provide an opportunity to reassess our medical priorities. Restrictions on bed supply should be accompanied by expansion of home ambulatory care programs and extended care facilities." The monotechnic view is not unknown among medical economists, but Mr. Fuchs, unlike some of his colleagues, understands where medical care has got to go: "Medical care performs other functions besides reducing morbidity and mortality," he says. "Particularly important are the caring function (sympathy, reassurance, relief of anxiety) and the validation function (provision of professional information about health status)."

When he finds out how to get physicians more concerned about these other functions, Mr. Fuchs can plant another flag, and crowds will cheer.

[1]Fuchs, Victor R., Who Shall Live? New York: Basic Books, Inc., 1974.

Notes on the Birth of the Blues

Amid the general confusion, the 50th Anniversary of pre-payment seemed a good time to remark the fact that some good things had happened.

April 1979

When the Blue Cross and Blue Shield Associations recommended that their member Plans should not pay for routine diagnostic tests for nonsurgical patients except when these are specifically ordered by physicians, thus in effect shrinking the familiar "admissions batteries" of laboratory procedures, the news appeared on page one of the *New York Times*. "Blue Cross-Blue Shield Moving to Curb Routine Hospital Tests," said the headline on a detailed story that took its place among reports of demonstrations in Iran, rising real estate values in Manhattan, a new $700 million federal housing project in the Bronx, and a Pakistani supreme court decision upholding the conviction of Zulfikar Ali Bhutto for complicity in a political murder. Pondering on how Blue Cross payments for chest X rays and urinalyses got to be world news, I was reminded of the time when, as a staff member of Chicago's Plan for Hospital Care, then a budding new enterprise that later became known as Blue Cross of Illinois, I accompanied the Plan director to a meeting of the medical staff of the old St. Luke's Hospital. The director had been invited to address the staff not because the doctors had expressed even the faintest interest in what he might say, but because the chairman of the hospital board of trustees, who was also a generous donor to its building and endowment funds, had been one of the organizers of the Plan and had made the arrangements.

It wasn't long before he wished he hadn't. As the director proceeded with his explanation of how the Plan was organized and what it hoped to accomplish, the mood of the doctors shifted from indifferent to inquisitive to doubtful to suspicious, and the questions that followed made it plain that some of them, at least, saw the new venture as an invitation to socialized medicine, if not revolution. When the meeting finally ended, the doctors were mutinous, the board chairman was furious, and I was dismayed. But the Plan director was unruffled. "Don't worry about it," he told me as we left the hospital. "Why, I can foresee a time when there will be Plans like ours in most of the cities—and there could be as many as a million members!"

I thought he was smoking opium—a feeling that I remembered distinctly last month as I read the *Times* story, which reported among other things that Blue Cross-Blue Shield now pays hospital and doctor bills for 112 million Americans.

How did it get that way? There must be reasons, and as the health insurance debate goes into rehearsal for the new season's performance, it may be instructive to consider what some of them are. One reason, certainly, is that right from the beginning, Blue Cross had its dedicated and talented crusaders. The one most celebrated at this year's 50th anniversary campfires is Justin Ford Kimball, the Texas school superintendent turned hospital administrator who is credited with putting the original model together at Baylor University Hospital in 1929.

The one group-one hospital Kimball model was quickly picked up and adapted for export. The exporters were an extraordinary group, totally unalike in background and talent but totally united in their zeal to carry the word to their communities. There was Frank Van Dyk, for example, a salesman and fund-raiser who never went beyond eighth grade but who figured out the actuarial base for the first communitywide Plans in New Jersey and New York and had the promotional gift to get them going and growing. E. A. van Steenwyk, a schoolteacher, writer, and editor, started the Plan in St. Paul, where he invented the Blue Cross, and later became director of the Plan in Philadelphia. Another pioneer, J. Douglas Colman, started with Van Dyk in New Jersey, then organized and directed the Plan in Maryland and later became president of New York Blue Cross. Still another was John Mannix, who had been interested in the prepayment idea as a hospital administrator in Elyria, OH, and later became a consultant to the Plan in Cleveland, then organized and ran the Plan in Detroit, where he negotiated the first

Blue Cross contract in the automobile industry. Mannix later directed the Plans in Chicago and Cleveland, but his most notable contribution may have been the auto contract, which has now endured for nearly 40 years and from the beginning included a medical service benefit sponsored by Michigan physicians on a model that had originated earlier in California. At the time, Mannix had envisioned a national coalition of hospital and medical plans, but as it turned out he was ahead of himself, and the national Blue Cross-Blue Shield network was developed only gradually over the course of the next several years.

Given the local community focus of the Plans and the individualistic, entrepreneurial character of their leadership, it may be astonishing that they ever did get together, and the fact that they did can be attributed largely to the efforts of Mannix, who kept on pushing the idea, and a man who was different from all the others in the same way a critic is different from an artist or performer. This was C. Rufus Rorem, a University of Chicago economist who had been a member of the staff of the national Committee on the Cost of Medical Care and of the Rosenwald Fund, a Chicago foundation for which he had undertaken a series of studies of hospital accounting and capital financing. This led to his appointment as chairman of the American Hospital Association's Committee on Uniform Hospital Accounting and, inevitably, involvement in the new group hospitalization prepayment movement. His articles on the subject began to appear in AHA and other publications in 1933. Three years later Rorem, with substantial backing from the Rosenwald Fund and enthusiastic acceptance by the AHA, became secretary of the AHA's Committee on Hospital Service, which evolved into the Commission on Hospital Service Plans and, eventually, the independent Blue Cross Association. Throughout the formative years it was Rorem who insisted on the principles that guided the early development and later growth of the Plans: not-for-profit organization, community service, public representation and supervision, and service benefits rather than cash indemnities. As Colman told an interviewer in 1971 when he was chairman of the executive committee of Blue Cross Association, "Rufus laid down the principles on which we operated and gave them visibility, credibility, and integrity."

Visibility, credibility, and integrity helped, but actually it took more than that to get Blue Cross and Blue Shield where they are today. It took an extraordinary confluence of the separate forces of industrial expansion, the rising strength of unions and industry-wide collective bargaining, the explosive advances of medical science and consequent specialization of medical practice in hospitals, the modernization and expansion of hospital facilities that had stood still during the years of depression and war, and the mounting awareness and expectations of a rapidly growing population. These currents were all flowing in the postwar years and the decades that followed, and the Blue Cross-Blue Shield concept provided a sort of unified field theory for the delivery of medical services, broadening and accelerating the rush of events and sweeping the Plans along with them. During these years, too, a new generation of Blue Cross-Blue Shield leadership was emerging, imaginative and idealistic like its predecessors but with an added dimension of the management skills demanded by vast enterprise and the flexibility to adapt Plan resources and experience to the requirements of new roles as intermediaries and carriers in Medicare. That this result was accomplished successfully following introduction of the Medicare program in 1966 and in the years since then has been verified repeatedly in HEW audits and in independent appraisals of intermediary and carrier performance. In fact, it is agreed on all sides that the Medicare contract has demonstrated an effective partnership of government and the private sector—a relationship that has evoked more bricks than bouquets in fields a lot less complicated than health care.

This isn't to say that it has been, or is now, or ever could be, smooth sailing. The unified field theory created excesses as well as successes, and in the present inflationary circumstances, worrying about the former has virtually silenced cheering about the latter. As is always the case when a problem obtrudes, in governments and corporations as in families, there is as much finger-pointing to assign blame as there is head-scratching to find answers, and in this case everybody is pointing at everybody else: hospitals are blamed for expanding too far and too fast, doctors for ordering too much too soon, Blue Cross and Blue Shield and insurance companies for covering too many services with too few constraints, unions for demanding benefits and corporations for providing them, government for overreaching with the new programs and then overreacting with regulations to curb them, consumers for overusing the whole system. There is probably some truth to all these allegations, but their endless repetition now tends to obscure the facts that half or more of the towering health care cost rise has been directly attributable to the general inflation that nobody knows how to or is willing to control, and a large part of the other half represents improvements in care that nobody wants to forego, and the cost of unnecessary services or abuses is a fraction that nobody can measure. Because the necessity of medical service is as much abstraction as reality, unnecessary services will never be completely eliminated, but they can be exposed and excised on occasion, and this is what the shouting is aimed at accomplishing.

Here everybody has a piece of the action, but it is uphill all the way because for most of the players the need to do less rather than more is a reversal of lifetime habits, as shocking to contemplate as it is for nations and corporations to consider that the time may come when growth can no longer be regarded as good per se. It is the disposition of the culture to equate more and better—no less for hospitals and doctors than for stores and states. Thus their voluntary efforts to suppress expenditures is in a way an unnatural act, like a bishop dancing, and their willingness to engage in it and suffer for it must be respected. So it is also for Blue Cross and Blue Shield, surely the most generous of insurers, whose voluntary cost containment effort is not new and includes revision of reimbursement practices, support for restrictive planning measures, encouragement of consultations in elective surgery, and now constraints on payment for diagnostic tests—all attempts to move upstream against the current that has been flowing so freely for 50 years. If the corporations and unions and consumers and congressmen and government agencies that have been so eager to jump all over the health care establishment would do as much to restrain their own excesses, we might at last have a grip on the inflation that threatens the whole society.

In any case, an anniversary is an occasion for celebration, not recrimination, and it wouldn't be a bad idea for hospitals and physicians to take time out this month for a thought to what Blue Cross and Blue Shield have accomplished in 50 years. It is customary at such moments, too, for the celebrants to look ahead and estimate the opportunities for the future. This is a chancy business always, and given the circumstance it is possible now to believe anything could happen. But it isn't too much to hope that with a little luck the kind of leadership and performance that made those St. Luke's Hospital doctors so wrong 50 years ago could keep them wrong for another 50 years.

This Is the Way It Was

November 1979

In ways unknown to the astrologists who tell us to take it easy and look for a surprise if we are Gemini or postpone long journeys if we are Taurus, the stars do indeed rule our lives, dividing time into rigid segments that dictate when we rise and retire, work and rest, worship and play, spend and pay, go forth and return. At times, the stars, and the contrivances we have devised to measure their turnings, tell us what to think about, as at the beginning of any day, week, month, or year we seek to envision the order of our activities with whatever hopes and fears our dispositions may allow, and at the end we look back with whatever satisfactions and regrets may be evoked. And especially now, when the stars move as always in their inverted bowl but our contrivances warn that they are about to mark off another decade, we are impelled to a surpassing ritual of remembrance and recapitulation. Ten years have passed, and we are bound to make an accounting to ourselves of what has been gained and lost. Unmindful that 10 years are passing every minute of every day, we are required by custom to make special measurements of where we have come from, preparatory to taking special soundings of where we are and special prophesies of where we are headed.

Ten years ago, then, our absorbing preoccupation was a war we hadn't wanted and had scarcely realized we were in until it had deposed an embarrassingly flamboyant but otherwise generally satisfactory president. We thought it was the war that had set the college campuses on fire, but a bright young acolyte of the deposed president had written a book about the student movement remarking that it was a worldwide phenomenon whose causes were rooted deeply in the social malaise. The war had lighted the fuse, but the dynamite had been in place long before, said the young man, whose ideas about the social malaise and what should be done about it were to become better known to the nation a little later on. His name was Joe Califano.

The stars moved, and the war was winding down—an expression we kept on using because it appeared to give the war a life of its own and remove us all another step away from having any responsibility for what happened. Whatever it was, another president got credit for it, for whatever that was worth, as he sought to cope with a threatening recession and a nagging inflation by giving us something that was called an Economic Stabilization Program because nobody wanted to call it wage and price controls. Along the way, a promised and promising family welfare program and family health insurance plan got lost, without much of anybody noticing that they had been around even momentarily. Before the ESP had run its three-year course, the entire nation had become transfixed by a political scandal that resulted, among other things, in a new word, a new president, a new awareness of the power of television, and what was called a new political morality but was actually just a new demonstration of what the state of political morality was and is. The scandal was also largely responsible for the fact that nobody realized how much the Economic Stabilization Program had really put the brakes on the inflation—the only time in the decade it happened that way.

Still, inflation was one of the problems the next president was confronted with. Another was national health insurance, which for 30 or 40 years had been an issue that wouldn't go away, and still is. The difficulty has always been that the must-haves and the can't-affords have never been able to resolve their intractable differences. They got part way there for old people and poor people in the 1960s, but Medicare and Medicaid have scared the can't-affords without satisfying the must-haves, so the standoffs persisted through the 1970s, and the issue is still with us.

But the issues that were overriding in the later years of the decade were inflation and energy. Still another new president told us early in what has been a turbulent presidential career that his energy program was the moral equivalent of war, but nobody knew what that meant, possibly including the new president, whose hortatory exertions have fallen short of moving the Congress to act on either of the major issues. For most of his term the president has insisted that the key instrument of his entire anti-inflation program has been the hospital cost containment bill, a strategy that told us more about the president's anti-inflation program than it did about hospital cost containment. But containment of the president's hard-core approach to hospital cost containment hasn't been easy. It has resulted partly from the early successes of the well-publicized effort to slow the inflation of health care costs organized by voluntary forces in the health care economy, and partly from well-organized lobbying by the same forces, which kept the bill in the bottle for two years and got it watered down with so many amendments that it wouldn't hurt much, or accomplish much, even if it were passed.

The fact is that it wouldn't do much good anyway. Trying to solve the inflation by suppressing one of its lesser results is like turning off the faucets while the house is being carried away in the flood. A critical cause of the inflation is the cost of energy, which is not soluble in either exhortation or politics, and very possibly not soluble at all, short of help from the stars. Meanwhile, the struggle to live with the results of inflation goes on. In the health care economy, the struggle has consisted principally of piling regulation on regulation to the point where confusion borders on chaos, and finally, some recognition that there must be a better way is emerging as the end of the decade is at hand. The better way seen by a few employers and insurers and professors, and a few even among the providers and regulators, would seek now to achieve an infusion of economic competition into transactions in which price has always been a nugatory consideration and the major components of choice have been availability, convenience, and either quality or satisfaction, depending on who's choosing. The proposed method, however, would require a massive injection of alternatives to the prevailing fee-for-service practice financed by insurance, and because nature hasn't produced enough prepaid group practices to create the desired degree of consumer choice, these would have to be manufactured synthetically. The process would have to be encouraged and, obviously, regulated by government, and protocols that have been prepared for inspection suggest that while the method might certainly be regarded as promising over time, it can scarcely be considered a substitute for regulation but would appear instead to offer the regulators a new playpen for their exercises.

An altogether different kind of better way was being tested increasingly in the late 1970s and gave some hope of taking the steam out of the health care cost inflation, but probably more hope to those who saw it simply as a means of improving the health status of the population—an old but sometimes forgotten value in medical care. This was known variously as the fitness mania, or the wellness movement, or, grandly, new directions in health care, and its proposition was simple enough: Make people healthier, and keep them that way, and they'll use less medical care and cost less. The movement had its theoretical origin early in the decade in England, where a group of physicians and other scientists deliberated at length and concluded that among all the factors contributing to the health of populations, notably including heredity, physical and social environment, occupation, and personal behavior, or life-style, as the new jargon had it, medical care was a lesser, and maybe the least, influence. Yet in most contemporary cultures medical care was where the greatest effort was concentrated. Some redress of investments was indicated, the savants recommended, but when the concept was transmitted to the United States some of its enthusiasts here got carried away and concluded that medicine wasn't worth that much anyway and needed to be put in its place. This expression was linked especially to the terms "holism" and "holistic medicine," which had a brief vogue but were applied indiscriminately to serious programs for considering the whole patient and all the influences on health, and to storefront metaphysicians promoting a wild potpourri of votaries and vibrations. Holistic medicine got a bad press and a bad name, and reputable doctors looked the other way.

But health promotion marches on, as anybody can tell by looking out the window. If the joggers aren't in sight, they will be in a minute, and the results of their earnest propulsion may eventually be measurable in improved cardiovascular and respiratory performance and diminished incidence of illness. For the moment, however, the score has been tallied mainly in the increased volume of visits to emergency rooms and doctors' offices for tendonitis, metatarsal disorders, and sagging uteri. Aches aside, the joggers are symbolic of an awakened national interest in health that is also apparent in changing diet practices, heightened awareness of health hazards in the environment, and the tendency of smokers to be either apologetic or belligerent about a habit that was taken for granted a decade ago. Alarmed about the amounts of money it was spending on employees' health insurance, industry joined the wellness movement with a variety of programs encouraging fitness and what is often called "health prevention"—a term whose internal contradiction is indicative of our genius for taking the meaning out of words. Corporate consultants are retained to screen employees to identify bad health risks and then refer them for treatment, or conduct classes and counseling for smokers, drinkers, compulsive eaters, and others whose life-styles are judged to be unhealthy and potentially expensive for employers. Nobody can prove yet that such programs pay off, but corporations have been willing to bet that they will.

So have hospitals, which have also picked up the health promotion signal and are intensifying their health information efforts for patients and families, and for their communities. In meetings, publicity, publications, and cooperative programs with public health departments, schools, and community groups, hospitals are organizing their considerable resources of knowledge and skills to motivate people to take more responsibility for their own health, and teach them how to stay well and how to make the most effective use of the services available to them when they get sick or hurt.

When the stars have whirled through their revolutions and turned up another set of observers to look back and remark the phenomena of this decade, however, it isn't likely that it will be the wellness movement, or the search for a new mode of practice, or the cost containment drive, or the regulatory havoc, or even the inflation, that will obtrude as the significant commitment of hospitals in the 1970s, so much as it will be the consolidation of independent units into multi-institutional organizations, or systems, as they are commonly called, though many of them have only the most rudimentary characteristics of the orderly arrangement suggested by the word. At the beginning of the decade, the hospital field was essentially a dispersion of discrete entities—joined together, to be sure, in regional, state, and national associations to share information and pursue common goals, but with few exceptions unattached to one another and uncoordinated in the management of their resources and the disposition of their services. By the end of the decade, an estimated 40 percent of the nation's hospital enterprise had coalesced in some 400 identifiable multiunit organizations having some formal cooperative agreement concerning their governance, management, operations, or services—or all or some of these. The terms of agreement varied all the way from loose arrangements for sharing plans and administrative services to central policymaking and management controls leaving only the details of day-to-day operations for local determination, and the experience suggested that the former might be expected to evolve toward the latter, as long as the central authority perceived and respected the values of local autonomy.

Either way, it was likely that the movement of freestanding hospitals into affiliations with others would continue, and it was estimated that as many as 75 percent of all hospitals would have joined some kind of multi-institutional system within a few years, moved not so much by any vision of improved service or efficiency as by the comforting shelter of a shield, or putative shield, against the invasive pressures of external circumstance. Not every hospital can afford a full-time lawyer, or even a full-time reader of the *Federal Register*, but every hospital today needs both. In the end, however, the multi-institutional systems, and the wellness business, and the new practice models, and the cost and regulation and inflation hassles, are less important than how well the doctors and hospitals perform their intrinsic tasks of caring for people who are sick and hurt. In the 1970s the distractions have appeared at times to be at center stage and the critical work of caring off in the wings, but this was an optical illusion that deceived only those who looked at the mirrored reflection of hospitals in headlines and politics instead of at the substance of hospitals in patients' rooms and corridors and doctors' workshops. The mirror may have misled some leaders in government and industry, and even some in the professions, but the real work of healing and comforting the sick goes on right along as it has in the past and will continue to do, as surely as the stars turn in the heavens. The stars and the healers are guided by the same Jurisdiction.

DOCTORS
AND DOLLARS

The Game Is About the Same

This is the way it looked at the beginning of the 80s. Two years later the outlook for change is a little stronger and the outlook for stability a little shakier, but the forces of tradition haven't been routed, and still aren't likely to be.

January 1980

For the greater part of the past decade it has been customary, if not compulsory, for hospital people to keep telling one another that "we are in a whole new ball game." In most cases the metaphor is a reference to the intervention of government in hospital affairs, and the incantation is in effect both a *nunc dimittis* for the good old days and a warning of horrors yet to come. Now I think that the practice of using sports analogs to describe social and political and business and professional phenomena has been pushed to the outer limits of credibility in our time, to the point where I have promised myself to get up and leave the room the next time anybody mentions a game plan, but my principal objection to the ball game trope is not that it is overused but that it is inaccurate. I don't think we are in a new ball game. We have some new rules, and some new players—and some of the new players are having trouble learning their positions. We also have some new methods of keeping score, and some new umpires whose interpretation of the rules many of us mistrust. But the game itself is about the same as it has always been, and from where I sit, in the press box, the chief difference is that the way it's being played today, nobody knows who has the ball.

The point is that the rules and the players have been changing right along and will continue to change, possibly at an accelerated rate, but we haven't yet thrown out all the players and started over, and we probably aren't going to. The guess

69

here is that at the end of the decade that is just beginning, the health care system is going to look pretty much the way it looks now. There will be more multiunit management systems, and more prepaid groups, and more government entitlements, which means more laws and more stringent regulations. And there unquestionably will be many new procedures and activities that nobody has thought of yet. But the basic components of the system will still be doctors and hospitals; the prevailing mode of practice will still be fee-for-service, and most of the hospitals will still be governed by voluntary boards of trustees and their professional managers—hemmed in by laws and rules even more than they are today but wielding the still considerable powers of local initiative and local autonomy and local professional and public support, rendered the more effective by decision and action in concert with other institutions and their associations.

There won't be as many hospitals at the end of the decade as there are now at the beginning. Already it is apparent that the principal method of controlling the number of beds, an inflexible obsession of rule makers who cling to the quaint notion that you can save the teacher's salary by taking empty desks out of the classroom, is not going to be planning boards, or utilization review, or even legislation or regulation per se, but withholding money. Laws and rules can be bent, but money that isn't paid can't be spent. By nibbling away at Medicare and Medicaid payments and dredging up and stretching a forgotton provision of a 35-year-old law, the Health Care Financing Administration, with assists from some of the states, has forced a few hospitals to close, and it seems inevitable that more will follow, and that nobody much except the voiceless workers and patients who are deprived of jobs and services will notice or care that more often than not the hospitals that close are those that are needed most, not least. If the closings that have occurred in the past year or two can be considered a foretaste of those to come, it is mainly densely populated inner-city neighborhoods and sparsely populated rural areas that will lose their hospitals. Ailing and injured old people and poor people will find their way to sources of care farther from home, if they can, and go without care if they can't. Either way, they will suffer most. They always do.

Elsewhere, the payment squeeze will compel a continued intensive search-and-destroy mission aimed at rooting out the inefficiencies that the authorities are convinced have been hiding under the beds. In some places some inefficiencies will be found and eliminated, unquestionably, as some already have been in the squeeze that is still largely voluntary. But the continuing money pressure will also compel many hospitals to discard some of the amenities that help ease the distresses of hospitalization for patients and families and add up to the patient satisfaction that is increasingly considered a component of high-quality care. Over time, chronic underpayment will erode the character of the professional environment and the performances of professional personnel, and invisibly but inexorably sap the quality of medical care at its core. This is what has been happening at many of our once great public charitable hospitals, deteriorated by years of overcrowding and underfunding. The process was described in a study prepared for the Commission on Public General Hospitals: "The affliction of the troubled inner-city public hospital is well known . . . obsolete buildings and equipment are poorly maintained; shortages of staff prevail at all levels, and labor unrest is ever present; critically ill patients are treated in a tense, crowded, and harried atmosphere; the quality of teaching programs is seriously compromised. Long waits in outpatient clinics are routine, and emergency rooms are jammed with patients in need of primary care who must wait their turn while emergencies are being treated."[1]

Could these things actually happen to any significant number of hospitals in the 1980s?

The public general hospitals that are threatened today have had a 50-year head start, and it isn't likely that many other hospitals are going to follow the path marked out by a generation of decline under local public authority management, payment policies, and politics. But the danger that rigidly imposed limits on payment could insidiously undermine quality is real, and so is the likelihood that the efforts to impose limits will continue. Safeguarding hospitals against encroachments on quality is thus seen as a principal function of hospital associations. "The anticipated efforts of state and local governments to trim spending and of the federal government to fight inflation and to protect the Medicare trust fund will combine to increase the pressures for hospital cost containment," said the American Hospital Association's "Environmental Assessment," the basic instrument for AHA's corporate planning.[2] "Concerted and sustained political action will be required to forestall deleterious legislation."

Many state and regional associations foresee the same course of events. "As costs continue to rise, government will try to turn hospitals into the whipping boy and enforce cost controls," James R. Neely, president of the Hospital Association of Pennsylvania, said. "While that will clearly not be very effective in the long run, in the short run it will cause us awful problems. This will make associations grow, for no hospital will be able to deal with that situation alone. I see a tremendous growth in associations in the 1980s. Where it occurs—national, state, or local—will depend largely on where the seat of government control over hospitals ends up." HAP vice-president John Russell summed it up: "Let's put a plaque out front saying 'Support bad government. It makes us grow."

David Kinzer of the Massachusetts Hospital Association agrees that income constraint is the overriding force making itself felt in hospitals, especially in the East, but he lists three other movements that will produce change at an accelerating pace in coming years. The others are the health planning act, which is creating an atmosphere where it becomes difficult for single hospitals to refuse to join forces, or look like they are joining forces, with their institutional neighbors; the fear of being too small; and the push for new approaches to financing. "The sabre rattling on the cost issue is most threatening to small hospitals," Kinzer said. "To be small is to be vulnerable, for a lot of reasons. Small hospital administrators [or, as it might be stated, administrators of small hospitals] are having more and more difficulty just coping with the floodtide of new regulatory demands pouring in on them. While they mostly still strive to maintain separate identity, many are now quietly but rather desperately looking for a mother."

The push for new financing methods can be seen as one result of the income squeeze, but it may also be something else, Kinzer suggested. "The big push for HMOs and other organizations that have provider risk-sharing as their theme is mainly a doctor game that our hospitals are watching apprehensively from the sidelines," he said. "For hospitals with soft occupancies, the new HMOs look like a potential solution to their problems, or, if not that, a main cause of their ultimate financial demise." And it is viewed by some as "the crumbling of the defense strategy of private fee-for-service medicine," he added. "It is getting easier to hire doctors on a salary, and the new physicians just out of their residencies are mostly looking for employment with organized medical groups." What it all adds up to, Kinzer concluded, is that "these four forces are the ingredients of major change in our business. Our boat is rocking. What we now have is the end of the status quo for our hospitals. We will always need and have hospitals, but they will be operating under different rules. If this is so, then state hospital associations, and for that matter all other hospital associations, must adjust to these rules or they can quickly become irrelevant."

It is possible to see the money crunch, the planning act, the impulse to seek solace in affiliation, and the HMO push as ingredients of major change without considering that they add up to a call for revolution and an end to fee-for-service medicine, or even a whole new ball game, but in any case it is plain that hospitals must comprehend and accommodate the new environment, and a look around among hospital associations suggests that helping the accommodation is already regarded as a central association function. As hospitals diversify their services and pursue expanding community roles, the need for a trusted entity to serve as information resource, negotiating forum, and industry advocate makes the association more important than it has ever been before, Pat Ludwig of the Michigan Hospital Association pointed out, but it also raises some questions about some of the operating programs that have been at the core of association service in past years—group purchasing, data processing, workers' compensation, professional liability, and many others that were pioneered by local, regional, and state associations and may now be challenged by the rapid formation of consortia, multi-institutional management systems, and chain operations offering similar capabilities. "We carried out a decade of shared services within a sister organization, and for all practical purposes have discontinued it," Elton TeKolste, president of the Indiana Hospital Association, said. "One reason these were no longer in demand was that our own hospitals are being encouraged to get into shared services and sharing their people with others."

Association executives for the most part are aware that changing external circumstance may bring shifts in emphasis among their representation, educational, and service functions, but nobody is predicting the early demise of association services; the outlook rather is viewed as pregnant with opportunity for new services—health education and promotion, expanded manpower training and recruitment, sponsorship and coordination of new enterprise such as ambulatory care centers, HMOs, home care, preventive services, and, especially, intensified advocacy. And association executives are by no means all agreed that chains and consortia are going to preempt established programs. "Anything they can do, we can do better" is the attitude of many, based on solid experience with large-scale purchasing and data processing programs, laundries, industrial engineering services, insurance plans, and management assistance functions of various kinds offering member institutions everything a consortium or management contract provides.

The thing associations can't provide is financial shelter, which can't be found in consortia or shared service arrangements, either, and this may foretell a period of accelerated merger, consolidation, and acquisition for hospitals. Some theorists argue that this is the only route to real economies in the system, anyway. Whoever is in charge, they say, management efficiencies at best can add up only to savings that are insignificant alongside those to be found in utilization controls, and controls affecting medical practice will never be effective as long as final authority resides in local governing boards that can be either intimidated, maneuvered, or persuaded by local doctors. Only when that authority is regarded as out of sight, out of reach, and formidable can rules governing utilization of facilities and services ordered by physicians begin to take hold, it is argued, and even then it is uphill work, as the PSRO experience has demonstrated.

The countervailing argument is that many local boards have been engaged effectively with their doctors to make utilization controls works, and these programs have been encouraged by the association-sponsored voluntary cost containment effort, which nearly everybody thinks will be continued indefinitely. Moreover, hospital associations almost without exception are initiating more educational programs for and more active participation by hospital trustees. Most of these are tilted toward intensifying trustee activity and influence in dealing with legislative and regulatory authority and coping with the financial pressures of the environment, but it is an interesting artifact of trustee education programs that no matter what subjects are listed in the agenda, the thing trustees want to talk about during the discussion periods and coffee breaks is doctors. And in contrast to the prevailing view of just a few years ago that the trustees worried about money and the doctors worried about patients, trustees increasingly understand today that the two are inseparable, and the task of the 1980s will be to get doctors to see it the same way.

Whether the heightened competition among health care services so devoutly promoted by critics of the present system, in and out of government, will tend to bring doctors and hospitals closer together or drive them farther apart isn't yet clear. You can get bets on either side, and the chances are it will go one way in some communities and the other way in others, depending on the nature and intensity of the competition, which is to say the number and composition of the HMOs that are seen as providing the competitive focus. In an interesting Delphi survey conducted among members of the board of trustees of the Illinois Hospital Association, most of them predicted that within the next five years "business will seek arrangements with particular hospitals to provide services for employees at an agreed price via HMO type arrangements."

If that should be the case, and if it turns out that events should move farther and faster along these lines than was foreseen earlier in this exercise, and hospitals start bidding against one another for HMO patients, with the low bidder getting the business, then the effect on the quality of care will be the same as that which could be expected to result from arbitrary limits on funding. Whether it is competition or regulation that is driving prices down doesn't matter in the end; the only difference would be that there are some communities that would be untouched by price competition and some hospitals that could remain aloof from the competition and survive, at least for a while, whereas regulatory limits would affect them all. But wherever it existed, price competition could be a threat to quality. An employer comparing bids on specified services from competing institutions might assume the lower bid was a better buy and have no way of finding out that the price difference in any case might represent different levels of skills and resources. Over time, competitive pressures could discourage hospitals from striving for excellence: Why risk having to raise the price and lose the business by buying new equipment, or hiring better trained technicians, or adding new services, when nobody would know the difference? The competition for excellence that exists now may result in some excesses that add to cost, but the price competition that is being urged on hospitals by economists and marketing geniuses from other fields would erode excellence, and cost more than money.

Nevertheless, the effort to inject price competition into the market for medical services is obviously going to be pursued; the fact that its effects could be disastrous in the absence of well known and easily understood methods of measuring quality will not dissuade or diminish the theological fervor of the faithful. But physicians are not as enchanted with the HMO model as professors and politicians have become, and employees are less concerned about cost than employers are, and, for the most part, are well satisfied with what they have. So it seems likely that the HMO injections will come in homeopathic rather than massive doses, allowing time for hospital associations to make headway with what has been an association function right along but is seen now as having surpassing importance for the coming decade—advocacy, or teaching legislators and bureaucrats and courts and employers and communities and the public how the system works. Especially, the need is for improving public understanding of the quality measures that already exist, as a protection against the chaos that would surely result if institutions, good and bad, should be pressured into advertising medical services like bath soap, as some of the marketing enthusiasts would have them do.

It must have been a sense of what may lie ahead that informed the Maryland Hospital Association's initiative in organizing a task force that spent a year or more examining the quality issue, and has now recommended establishment of a Maryland council for quality health care, described as a kind of state level Institute of Medicine, or independent scientific body, whose function would be to define and interpret measures of quality and help resolve the public questions of quality in relation to cost that seem certain to become the critical health care issue of the 1980s. As proposed, the council would be governed by a board selected for the scientific integrity and public credibility of its members and thus free of the suspicion of bias that attaches to judgments or rulings handed down from professional, institutional, and political sources. Whether or not the pronouncements of such an independent body would be heeded by legislators and public rate approval authorities remains to be seen, but providers, employers, consumers, and insurers would be bound to pay attention, and the presence of a visible and credible center of quality information should put some constraints on the zeal to drive cost down at the expense of quality, on one side, and the tendency to plead quality as a screen for excess or inefficiency, on the other. With a little luck, it might also tend to keep the competition honest. After spending a lifetime in the highly competitive publishing business, I can testify that keeping the competition honest is not something that happens by itself. It is ironic, not to say tragic, that the Federal Trade Commission—the agency of government we depend on to keep competition honest—is one of the forces pushing hospitals, whose keen competition for excellence in the past has been as clean as you can get, into the kind of price competition that is most likely to get dirty.

Associations elsewhere have shown interest in the Maryland concept, and if it can be made to work it will surely be adapted—perhaps most usefully in metropolitan areas, where the concentration and diversity of physicians, hospitals, employers, insurers, and consumers can be expected to create the most intensive competitive pressures and the most urgent need for dispassionate adjudication. Moreover, if the independent council model helps the public to sort out the entangled values of cost and quality, it might also address the moral issues that will weigh more and more heavily on physicians, administrators, trustees, and their associations as limitations on resources collide increasingly with public expectations and demands in the 1980s. Already there is rationing of high-technology care for the terminally ill and the prematurely born; the dispositions are made largely within institutions and without schemata. But as resources and demands abrade, affecting a widening segment of the population, institutions will be compelled to address the moral complexities of developing systems for determining who shall have care. Up to now, when the question of rationing care has come up, physicians and hospital administrators have insisted that they shouldn't have to make the decisions. "The society must decide," they like to say. But society's decisions are always crude and often cruel. For large segments of the population the answer to "Who shall live?" in the past has been "Who can pay?" The new entitlements have cut down the numbers excluded from care by that crude standard, and even in what promises to be a decade of austerity, some new entitlements are expected.

But the question now isn't just who shall live, or who shall get care. It is also what kind of care, and how much, and for whom. Inevitably, these are in part economic questions, and in part political. But at root there are also moral issues, and hospital trustees and administrators and associations couldn't do any greater service for the society than they can do by teaching and emphasizing the moral dimension of quality in medical care and insisting that the moral values should be considered and weighed along with the other components of quality, and the economic and political values that obtrude. If consideration of quality, including the moral dimension, should get lost among the competitive pressures of the 1980s, and medical services are advertised and sold like soap, it won't make much difference what institutions and associations do, because nobody will believe them.

[1]O'Rourke, P.F., The Inner-City Public Hospital: Challenges and Options. Readings on Public General Hospitals, prepared for the Commission on Public General Hospitals. Chicago: Hospital Research and Educational Trust, 1978.

[2]American Hospital Association, Environmental Assessment of the Hospital Industry, 1979, Chicago: AHA, 1979.

Too Many One-Eyed Critics

December 1977

In a year in which the President has publicly declared hospital costs to be an urgent national problem, the Secretary of HEW has repeatedly described the hospital industry as obese, congressmen have leaped over one another in their eagerness to introduce bills aimed at curbing the hospital inflation, and the nation's editorial writers and cartoonists have wrung out their adjectives and animosities picturing hospitals as extravagant and uncaring, it isn't surprising that some hospital people have lashed back in anger at the public critics as uninformed and unfair. Others, shaken by the ferocity of the onslaught, look around for somebody else to blame, and there is no great shortage of candidates. Among those nominated to share the scapegoat role are unions, health insurers, consumers, regulators, suppliers, the press, and hospital industry leaders themselves, who are charged by some with failure to create an adequately benign public understanding of the intricacies of hospital costs.

Given an industry that might readily be seen as seething with dissension in the relentless glare of public discontent, why isn't it giving off sparks like a sputtering fuse? Why do only a handful of its members write indignant letters to editors blaming everybody but themselves? When an insurance executive said at a recent meeting that the entire health care system is teetering on the brink of total collapse, why was it the hospital administrators in the audience, and not the physicians or educators or government officials or businessmen, who pointed out that he didn't know what he was talking about? Certainly it isn't because hospital administrators are either brighter or dumber than the rest of the population. Like physicians and bureaucrats and congressmen and industrialists and pipefitters and housewives, hospital people come in all sizes, shapes, and kinds. Some of them are tall and some are short, some are cheerful and some

79

gloomy, some sharp and some dull, some wise and some foolish. But all of them are obviously aware that they and their institutions are the prime targets for restrictive legislation and the chief focus for the concerns of industry, insurers, unions, and consumer organizations with the costs of health care. How is it, then, that the hospital industry, like Kipling's hero, seemingly can keep its head when all around it are losing theirs?

Granted that it doesn't require an advanced form of sanity to look good alongside public officials shouting obesity and insurance executives crying calamity, there are good reasons for believing, as most hospital people do, that the industry will still be here when the smoke clears or will keep on operating in the smoke if it doesn't clear, which it might not do. The most obvious reason is that it is the first responsibility of everybody inside the health care industry, often overlooked by everybody outside, to take care of people who are sick and hurt. To be sure, the zealous pursuit of this goal may result in excesses and on occasion has been used as a screen to hide inefficiencies. But it is a libel of the system to insist, as has been done, that excess and inefficiency, and not concern for patient care, are the rule, and the reason hospital people can avoid panic in the face of the libel is that it is patently untrue, as one million hospital patients on any day would rise to testify. So would the thousands of voluntary donors, great and small, who contribute each year $5 billion or more to the nation's hospitals—not notably a vote of no confidence. Among all the voices raised to censure hospitals, the voices of hospital patients are strikingly absent, save for only an occasional complaint about a rude or indifferent doctor or nurse or attendant. More often than not, these lapses are unnoticed or shrugged off as inconsequential by hospital administrators unless there is reason to suspect incipient liability, in which case defensive maneuvers may be initiated. Actually, any such episode is a distortion of mission that should require investigation and remedial action. But the point here is that at worst these occurrences are infrequent and can scarcely be considered grounds for condemning three million hospital employees. The complaints about cost also come from everybody but patients. Economists like to point out that the reason this is so is that patients don't have to pay the bills themselves at the time they are sick, because most of the bills today are paid by insurers and government agencies. The argument would be a lot more persuasive if people were all as dumb as economists think they are and didn't know they were paying for the insurance and government programs.

Another reason the hospital industry is relatively calm under fire is that the public uproar, as Mark Twain once said of Wagner's music, isn't really as bad as it sounds. In fact, it isn't really public. It doesn't come from the public, which is an abstraction anyway, but from the various kinds of elected and appointed and self-appointed public surrogates who buy or bargain for, or concern themselves with, health care services on behalf of the populations they represent, or think they represent. The surrogates are all the members of Congress and the state legislatures, the health program directors and assistant directors and assistant assistants in all of the various public agencies, the prepayment and insurance executives, the employers and union leaders and consumer organizers, and the subspecies of all these species, who are making so much noise that they can't hear the silence of their constituencies, or putative constituencies. The hospital industry hears the silence and knows what it means. It means the people aren't all that dissatisfied with what they're getting, even at today's prices. Some public opinion geniuses dispute this and insist that their polls show rising public concern about hospital costs, but it isn't clear whether this is cause or effect. It may be that the repeated image of governors, senators, cabinet members, and lesser types moaning in Macy's window rubs off on the rest of us to the point where expressing no worry about hospital costs would be considered doltish. Thus doom multiplies itself in our time.

The surrogates are not stupid, however, and it seems likely that their uproar, which might be called semipublic uproar, is going to accomplish something. There will be some economies that might not have come about without the uproar, such as those that may result from the movement to shared services, and consortia, and multiunit management systems. These phenomena have been around for years, but there can't be much question that their development has been accelerated by external pressures, including the pressure to get inside the stockade before the Indians attack. Some excesses of building and equipment will be avoided and some overreaching of staffing and services diminished by the prodding, too, and some "shrinkage of the system" accomplished—to use the new idiom that likens a $150 billion industry to a Chinese laundry. All these can be put down as gains by those who are counting, but there will be some countervailing losses. Some patients will be comfortless in drafty old buildings that Surrogate A has condemned as obsolete while Surrogate B says they can't be replaced because there are too many beds on the other side of town, and some patients will get short shrift as staffing ratios are shaved to keep budgets within limits set by Surrogate C. Some doctors are going to walk out of their hospitals because Surrogate D says they can't have a new scanner, or whatever; the doctors will go across the street and buy one for their offices, outside Surrogate D's jurisdiction, and then to accommodate the patients they take away from the hospital they'll duplicate more of the hospital's equipment. Only a one-eyed view could see this as shrinking the system. The problem is the incidence of one-eyed surrogates.

Whether the gains outweigh the losses or not will depend on who is doing the measuring, because there isn't much agreement on which is which. Either way, it isn't only the hospitals and doctors and insurers and public surrogates who will decide the way things go. It never has been. The view that for the past 30 years the people have been manipulated by some hospital-medical-money establishment into buying a system they didn't need and didn't want is a myth born of the need for a scapegoat to share the blame for inflation, cognate with the theory that the society didn't really want all those automobiles it has been buying over all those years, or all the highways and high rises and mobile homes and plastic swimming pools. It is true that supply creates demand to a greater extent in the market for medical services than is the case in other markets, but the growth of the hospital industry couldn't have happened unless the people wanted it that way, and it is going to keep on happening, though unquestionably at a somewhat subdued pace, in spite of all the brakes that may be applied. The only thing that can really shrink the health care system is a depression. This is a possibility that has to be comprehended, but not while the brakes are being fixed.

Meanwhile, there are some powerful forces pushing for more. One is constantly rising public expectation, which doesn't show many signs of turning around and going the other way, in spite of the sudden surge in the number of people who feel impelled to run five miles before breakfast, eschew cigarettes, eat bran, and count their triglycerides. These and other indications that people are becoming more willing to share the responsibility for their own health are seen by some as evidence that the society may be turning away from medicine, but it isn't a cause for rejoicing yet. Half the joggers are going to require foot or knee surgery in middle age, for one thing, and, for another, the total population of new health seekers is only a tiny fraction of the population whose cancer and heart disease are yet to come, gifts of the industrial polluters of our airs, waters, and foods, who get an occasional rap on the knuckles from the surrogates who can spare time from beheading the hospitals.

Another force to be weighed is the new technology that will inevitably continue to emerge and be deployed, and in fact demanded. Consider what would happen, for example, if one or another of the hundreds of hypertension research laboratories around the country should suddenly come up with a new medication, more effective than all the others, that would require a few days of hospitalization, as is done now in diabetes, to work out individual dosage requirements and stabilize treatment. There are an estimated 24 million Americans suffering from hypertension. Still another thing that has to be considered is the changing composition of the population. The World Health Organization has projected that the percentage of the population over age 65 may rise as much as 50 percent over the next generation, and as we know, this swelling segment requires three or four times as much health care as the rest of the population does. And it isn't all nursing homes, foot massage, and strained soup. The aged need more high technology care too: organ repair and replacement, surgery and radiation and chemotherapy for neoplasms, and the new and exciting rehabilitation aids.

I want to be in that number when the saints go marching in to the HSA meetings with their computers and their guidelines, and discover that the people most opposed to cutting down beds and rejecting applications for equipment are not the doctors and nurses and hospital administrators but all those consumer representatives on the boards. When that happens, the thing that is going to collapse isn't the health care system. It's the regulatory system.

Where National Policies Come From

July 1978

Like a well-kept garden, the health care conference can be expected year after year to produce a suitable display of bright, fragile blossoms springing from new seeds of thought, along with the perennials that emerge in season with texture and color unchanging from year to year and roots deeply embedded in the soil of conventional wisdom. Perhaps the liveliest of the new blooms that appeared in this conference season have been marketing, patient education, and the voluntary cost containment effort—all favorites whose new tints and fragrance were attractive. But new ideas can be troubling, and conference audiences were relieved on occasion to turn to such reliable, recurring themes as regulation, finance, utilization, management, quality assurance, and public policy, where all sides could agree, as they have been doing now for years, that the underlying problems are not anybody's fault, actually, so much as they are the result of the fact that we lack a national health policy. Given clearly formulated goals and policies directed toward achieving them, the argument runs, national priorities can be established and all these problems of cost, access, utilization, and finance can be sorted out and addressed. Once this is said, since it can be assumed that nobody is going to be articulating national health policy, we can relax and continue hacking away at the problems as they present themselves, each institution or organization or profession in its own fashion.

Is this really the case? Do we indeed lack a national health policy, and is this a barrier to resolution of the many difficulties that beset the nation's health services? Or is the putative lack of policy more nearly a comfortable myth screening all the separate interests from the need to face up to their differences one by one as a necessary step toward formulation of a coherent system?

It can be argued with some logic that the trouble may be too much health policy, not too little. Certainly we have a national health policy, as well as programs, for example, for the aged and the poor, for the disabled and the medically indigent, for mothers and infants, and for sufferers from renal disease. We have a national health policy too for members of the armed forces and their dependents, for veterans and federal employees, for native Americans and migrant workers. There is national policy governing income tax deductions for medical and health insurance expense, and for that part of the population that is untouched by any of these policies, the policy for the moment is that there is no policy, except as the entire population in one way or another is affected by national policy concerning health facility construction and health planning, biomedical research and quality assurance, health manpower and education, and by policy for drugs and devices, foods and cosmetics, radiation and environment, and occupational hazards. If it is considered that we must have a single national health policy, then it would have to be the sum of all these discrete health policies—but look quickly now, because the parts keep shifting and the sum will not be the same tomorrow.

Of course, this is just the point. Instead of a single, coherent, directed national policy with clear goals suggesting courses of action, we have this gallimaufry of policies all over the place, diverging and at times colliding, and changing with the temperatures of the appropriations committees. It would be tidier to have a single, coherent policy by which all concepts and programs could be guided and measured, but anybody who thinks this is likely to happen, now or at any time, has only to consider how any one of the existing health policies was developed.

For example, national health insurance for the aged and the poor might be thought of as a latter-day creation of the liberal, and some say extravagant, 89th Congress, obedient to President Lyndon Johnson's vision of a Great Society, and it is a fact that the entitlements were indeed enacted by that Congress, not unmindful of that stimulus. But that Congress wasn't unmindful either of the long history of national health insurance policy discussions in the United States, which began in earnest with studies of sickness insurance in Europe by a special committee of the American Medical Association before World War I. The committee was impressed by the need for and inevitability of some form of medical insurance for Americans, as it turned out, and its recommendations moved the AMA, briefly and stormily, in that direction.

Then the concept of national health insurance disappeared from public view for a few years. It emerged again in 1932 in the report of a prestigious national Committee on the Cost of Medical Care, whose recommendations caused rioting in hospital corridors. As a consequence, medical insurance was dropped from President Franklin Roosevelt's social security program before the Social Security Act was passed by the Congress in 1935, and there are those today, possibly including some in the AMA, who think we might be better off if he had dropped the Old Age and Survivor's Insurance and kept the health insurance. But the point here is that national health insurance didn't die; it just went underground again for a few more years of depression and then war. Health insurance bills were introduced in the Congress during those years but were not taken seriously again until after the reelection of President Harry Truman in 1948, when an insurance proposal once more became a public issue. This one also faded, in part because of continued strong opposition, and in part because of public preoccupation with the Korean War. But the intervals were getting shorter. In the 1950s, the health insurance issue came to focus on the elderly, whose special needs for help were obvious to everybody, although there was little agreement on what direction the effort to meet them should take. But there were growing numbers who became convinced that legislation mandating assistance would be required, and in 1960 the Congress, after rejecting several other proposals, passed the Kerr-Mills Act providing federal grants to states for medical payments to old age public assistance recipients and aged persons not on public assistance but unable to pay medical bills.

But Kerr-Mills proved to be too little, too late, and soon the debate heated up again as the Congress and interested segments of the population considered new entitlements in the friendlier environment of a new federal administration. By the time the Social Security Amendments of 1965 were passed, including Medicare and Medicaid, the national health policy represented in the legislation had been in the making for 50 years, and nobody in his right mind can believe that the process stops here.

The Social Security Amendments of 1972, which gave us such loaves and fishes as PSRO and section 1122, had a similar, if less tortuous, history. Utilization policy, now embedded in PSRO, can trace its ancestry back to 1913, when Dr. E.A. Codman developed his system of outcome measurements for surgical patients at the Massachusetts General Hospital and was thrown out of office by his local medical society for his pains. Then as now, however, physicians dedicated to medical care evaluation were an indomitable lot, and Dr. Codman not long afterward was assisting at the birth of the American College of Surgeons and its Hospital Standardization Program, which begat the Joint Commission on Accreditation of Hospitals. JCAH became the uncle, if not the parent, of the utilization review provisions of Medicare, which were observed more in form than in substance—a default that brought us first EMCRO and then PSRO, which has had a few outstanding successes but whose record on the whole may have Dr. Codman wondering if he was on the right track. Either way, it doesn't seem sensible to conclude that PSRO is the end of the line for utilization policy.

The concept of regionalization of health facilities and services has been around ever since Aesculapius established his temples of healing at Cos, Epidaurus, Cnidus, and Pergamos, and, in fact, specific catchment areas for specific institutions have been the rule rather than the exception in the development of hospital systems everywhere except in America, where the whims of philanthropists and the convenience of surgeons, rather than the logic of geography and economics, generally dictated sites and services. The Committee on the Cost of Medical Care had something to say about regionalization, but nobody was building anything in 1932 and, besides, the committee's health insurance recommendations made all its conclusions suspect. The Lanham Act of 1942 providing federal funds to help build hospitals and schools in "defense impacted areas," as they were delicately called, was a glimmer of things to come in planning. A National Commission on Hospital Care in 1946 envisioned regional linkages of rural health stations, small hospitals, larger institutions for larger communities, and, finally great medical teaching centers for great populations—all these, it was postulated, joined and integrated by rational referral and educational practices. The same vision fueled passage of the Hill-

Burton Act the same year, but the vision was quickly dissipated as Hill-Burton funds were administered in large part according to the demands of local physicians, local money, and local pride, rather than regional need.

These are formidable forces, still very much in evidence. They made the Comprehensive Health Planning and Partnership for Health and Regional Medical Program Acts of 1966 and 1967 into largely ineffective gestures as voluntary planning boards went through the motions of approving one another's projects, and it isn't by any means certain that the consumer majorities on the boards of the Health Systems Agencies created by the National Health Planning and Resources Development Act of 1974 are going to be that much more effective. When consumers have been strong or willful enough to reject expansion plans backed by professionals on HSA boards, and it hasn't happened every day, more often than not the board decisions have been overturned by recourse to political muscle. Regional rationalization of the health care system is obviously desirable, and it is not likely to be abandoned as health planning policy. Unfortunately, it collides with another policy that has even deeper roots in American life: local autonomy. Up until now, it would appear that the policy that got there first has always had the stronger arm.

This sketchy account of the development of just three of the fragments that add up to national health policy as it now exists suggests some of the complexities from which policies emerge, slowly but not finally, as the product of contending forces. And this account has considered chiefly the legislative component of policy making, but it is well known that the executive and judicial branches may have a hand, and sometimes the upper hand, in determining the course of events. Thus, utilization policy today may owe more to *Darling* than to the Senate Finance Committee, and the folklore of the 1960s had it that it was a knowledgeable Secretary of Health, Education and Welfare, and not the Great Society concept, that made Medicare and Medicaid a reality. Moreover, we are persuaded at times that it is not the visible senators and audible secretaries who have the most influence in shaping policies, but the lesser bureaucrats and staff members, some of whom have been known to do most of the thinking and writing that become laws, and rules, and policies. The process was described in a recent article about the

Assistant to the President for National Security Affairs, and it can probably be assumed that foreign policy, which seems at least as fragmented, incoherent, and multidirectional as health policy, results in much the same way. "One staff member told me recently," the author related, "'I spend all my time on one area, and I realize that I skim off only a tiny percentage of what I should know. There are at least 200 or 300 items a day in my in-box. I have to sort out what it's essential for Brzezinski and the President to know. When I think of how hard it is for me to stay on top of things, I have to believe that it's impossible for the President, Vance, and Brzezinski.'"[1] Remarking his inability to move the relatively lean bureaucracy of his time to his way of thinking, President Roosevelt complained that dealing with the permanent government establishment was like punching a paper bag. Other Presidents have described the same phenomenon in more vigorous language, and President Carter just recently worried in public about "the iron triangle of bureaucracy, Congressional committees, and well-organized special interests." Even Presidents, it appears, are frustrated for want of clear, coherent national policy.

It is not comforting to reflect that national health policy, or foreign policy, or economic policy may be determined in some part by what an anonymous assistant's assistant thinks is important or not important for his chief, and his chief's chief, to see. But it is not sensible to think that it could be any other way. Since this is the case, it is unquestionably a good thing that important policies like national health insurance and health planning and utilization have been 50 years in the making and are still evolving by the painful process of rubbing the information, experience, interests, opinions, and biases of Presidents, secretaries, senators, nameless assistants, professions, institutions, and consumers against one another until something resembling policy may be extruded. The process is woefully cumbersome and inefficient, and it isn't ever going to produce a single, coherent, directed national health policy with clear goals suggesting courses of action. But it is a marvelous protection against error, and against sudden shifts in direction. So long as we cling to this abrasive, fragmented, inefficient method, we shall avoid the danger of clearly articulated coherent, directed national health policy—laid down by a single person or group or interest, and wrong. If secretaries made policy, for example, we might now have a national health policy forbidding smoking. It might be good for the nation's health, but it would be a hell of a way to run the country.

[1]Drew, E., A Reporter at Large, (Brzezinski), The New Yorker, 54:70; May 1, 1978.

Bureaucracies Don't Die— Or Even Fade Away

David Kinzer's book is out of date now, and the bureaucracies he wrote about are under siege—but they're still there, for the reasons suggested here.

September 1977

Forty years ago, give or take, an Italian Marxist scholar named Bruno Rizzi predicted in a book called *The Bureaucratization of the World* that bureaucracies would become the new ruling class, telling polictical authorities what they could and couldn't do, instead of the other way around, which is the way things have generally, if not unexceptionally, worked out. Rizzi thus turned the tables on Karl Marx, who had considered bureaucracies an instrument of the ruling class that would wither and vanish with the advent of the classless society—an eventuality that has eluded us for the first 100 post-Marx years and looks good to stay out of reach for as far ahead as anybody can see now. Still another celebrated scholar of bureaucracy, the German sociologist Max Weber, said bureaucracies were permanent and indispensable and would prevail in governments, armies, universities, and churches. The trick, according to Weber, would be to maintain a balance or tension of bureaucratic and political autonomies; if either were to become dominant, he thought, the society or organization would be destroyed. An earlier student of the subject, John Stuart Mill, the British economist and utilitarian philosopher, who spent 30 years as a clerk and department head for the East India Company and later became a Member of Parliament and thus had ample opportunity to observe the species in its native habitat, wrote in 1861 that "Bureaucracy accumulates experience, acquires well tried and well considered maxims, and makes provision for appropriate practical knowledge in those who have the actual conduct of affairs. But it is not equally favorable to individual energy of mind," he added, delicately calling attention to a quality that has been described on occasion in more colorful language. Like Weber, Mill thought the excesses of bureaucracies would destroy their organizations. "The disease which afflicts bureaucratic governments, and which they usually die of, is routine," he wrote. "They perish by the immutability of their maxims."

Obviously, it takes a while. The government Mill wrote about is still around, having survived wars, strikes, depressions, decolonizations, and reforms that would have been called revolution if the bloodshed had been visible, and it is possible to believe that Mill was wrong and the immutability of the maxims, as much as the individual energy of mind of those who have the actual conduct of affairs, is a stabilizing force that keeps governments going in spite of the periodic upheavals that afflict them all. The characteristics of bureaucracy that give continuity to enterprise have been recognized since the time of Plato's Republic, which had its class of guardians who carried on the business of the state. These characteristics were listed by Weber, among others, as an authority structure or, in the language of sociology, pyramidal hierarchy, a system of specialized tasks and individual roles, and a system of control based on prescriptive principles or rules. As Weber pointed out, these are the characteristics of armies, churches, and universities, as well as governments, and ever since the industrial revolution these have also been the characteristics of industrial and business corporations. Mill's East India Company was an early example; it had not only bureaucrats but a college in London where they were trained—possibly the ancestral home of the graduate schools of business, whose students are taught the art of climbing pyramidal hierarchies to their peaks. It is an irony of our time that the bureaucrats of business commonly despise the bureaucrats of government, not understanding that their chromosomes look about the same under the microscope.

One of the graces of this account of bureaucratic misadventure by David Kinzer[1] is that beneath his understandable frustration at the inconsistencies and injustices of the regulatory labyrinth that is threatening to suffocate the hospital industry, one can glimpse his perception that the regulators, too, are victims, compelled by laws and circumstances they did not create to make rules for an industry whose power is generated by forces outside the jurisdiction of its own bureaucracies. So long as lawmakers seek means to control the industry without laying hands on the physicians who furnish the fuel for its engines, the rulemakers must continue to write gibberish. Not everybody understands this—including some at the peaks of the hospital pyramids. Meanwhile, Kinzer may have found the only solution consistent with preserving sanity: He stopped reading the gibberish.

One thought will occur again and again to all who read this book—to hospital administrators, who will read it with all the fascination of one who examines a cut to watch it bleed; and to trustees, who may thus enlarge their grasp of the complexities they must cope with somehow; and to physicians, who already are beginning to feel the effects of the rule-making and should understand what lies ahead, and to government officials and lawmakers, who are all familiar with some of the parts but may find here a new perspective of the whole—all these will ask themselves over and over, "Does it really have to be this bad?" Kinzer thinks not, and his two dozen proposals for reform are aimed for the most part at consolidating agencies, integrating state and federal controls, addressing regulations to demand as well as supply sources, and facing up to the obvious need for some involvement of physicians that will modify the impact of their decisions on hospital utilization and expense without invading their freedom. Kinzer doesn't know how this can be done, and neither does God. "The tangled mess that I have described in this study is the result of legislative bodies trying to address a whole lot of health problems on an *ad hoc* basis, and then regulators trying to codify, administer and enforce the laws," he concludes. "It seems too much to expect that these same people can gather up this whole bag of confusion and, with just a few new laws and new regulations, produce something coherent. This is not the way the system works. This suggests that the rationalization of health regulation must be achieved through persistent lobbying from the outside. The lobbying can't be just *ad hoc* resistance to new health laws and regulations but must derive from a strategy that takes a systems approach to a very large, complex, and frightening problem."

That isn't going to happen either, not for want of persistent lobbying but for want of a strategy. Unlike the oil industry, or the lumber industry, or one or two others where a handful of huge corporations all want the same thing and know just what it is and don't care what happens to the rest of the industry and so have a strategy, the hospital industry consists of thousands of units ranging in scale from General Motors to the corner bicycle shop and is so mission-oriented that the industry is equally concerned for both and the only thing they all want is to be let alone, and that isn't a strategy. It isn't even a hope. The configuration of the industry is changing, to be sure, with more units in chains or management systems, more mergers, more shared services and joint enterprises and consortia, and it is possible that another generation of bureaucrats may be able to write prescriptions that can curb some without killing others. But by that time there will be 40 million people over age 65 and standing room only in hospitals and the drive will be to get beds built, not tear them down. But if most physicians are still in private fee-for-service practice, and they may be, and if the lawmakers still consider that they mustn't lay hands on white coats, and they may still think so, then this tangled mess that Kinzer describes here may not be all that different, unless perhaps it is worse.

It seems certain to get worse before it can get any better as the federal government shapes up its plan to lay a flat ceiling on increases in payments to all kinds of hospitals for all kinds of patients, a stricture whose details and regulations are going to make the rules for planning and utilization review and eligibility and reimbursement that Kinzer has described look as simple as Dick and Jane. Under the circumstances, the blood pressures of hospital administrators and trustees seem certain to be dangerously elevated, and it is possible that even Kinzer, whose report is notably good natured in tone, considering its content, may be moved from incredulity to indignation. The target of most of the wrath will be bureaucrats, but is is likely, again, that the bureaucrats will be more victims than culprits and more to be pitied than cursed. Decisions like this are made by those who have the actual conduct of affairs, who generally haven't been around long enough, and usually don't stay around long enough, to know what the problems are, much less the answers. This is not a new phenomenon of government. John Stuart Mill said in his famous essay on representative government that "the interests dependent on the acts done by a public department, the consequences liable to follow from any particular mode of conducting it, require for weighing and estimating them a kind of knowledge, and of specially exercised judgment, almost as rarely found in those not bred to it, as the capacity to reform the law in those who have not professionally studied it."

It may be that the most effective strategy for the hospital industry today would be persistent lobbying to get Kinzer's report into the hands, and heads, of as many as possible of those who have the actual conduct of affairs, in Washington and the states, so that they might thus be helped to know the consequences liable to follow from any particular mode of conducting a public department. Until this can be done, the immutability of the bureaucratic maxims may help as much as it hurts.

[1] Kinzer, D., Health Controls Out of Control, Chicago: Teach'em, Inc., 1977.

What's Good for General Motors

August 1978

In one of the early exhibitions of industry's concern about the high cost of health services, Motorola, Inc., or one it its executives, became exercised several years ago about what were seen as inefficiencies or extravagances in the operation of hospitals in Phoenix, AZ, where the corporation had several thousand employees. Not all the hospitals were eager to comply with Motorola's requests for information about hospital operations and finances, and, in the fashion that sometimes makes the trend toward public disclosure seem a mixed blessing, what began as a technical disagreement between parties of divergent perspectives quickly became a burning public issue. It was resolved, eventually, without lasting damage on either side. Some hospital practices were modified, the intensity of Motorola's involvement subsided, and that part of the public that pays any attention at all to the antics of the Samaritans may have learned something about both hospitals and corporations.

Nevertheless, the Motorola episode was more beginning than end. Industry's dismay about health care costs became national news not long afterward when it was reported that General Motors paid more for employees' health care than it did for steel. Actually, what GM had said was that it had paid more to Blue Cross-Blue Shield, the major supplier of health insurance for GM employees, than it had paid to United States Steel, the major supplier of steel for GM cars. But the company's protests that it really pays a lot more for steel than it does for health care got lost among the headlines and never caught up with the more compelling version, and it doesn't really matter anyway, because the fact is that GM is concerned enough about the amount the company is paying for health care to have initiated its own voluntary cost containment effort, a broad program that includes restructuring the insurance coverage wherever changes can save money without damaging care; conducting studies and experiments in medical necessity review, preadmission testing, second surgical opinions, and prospective reimbursement; and a number of activities in early detection and prevention of disease and insafety and health education. The reason General Motors is obtruding its blunt industrial bumpers into these and other recondite professional matters was stated simply by Victor Zink, director of employee services and benefits. "Our monthly cost for each covered employee and retiree and their families averages about $134. This is an increase of 50 percent over the last three years. Practically none of this increase was related to improvements in benefits."

Speaking at a meeting of hospital financial managers, Zink readily acknowledged that industry is not without some responsibility for cost escalation. "As our critics tell us, we are partly to blame because of our excessive insurance coverages," he said, "but all elements of the health care system have contributed to the problem as well. Through the years, we did what we thought best under the circumstances. People wanted hospital beds, so we built them. People wanted more doctors, so we educated them. People wanted first dollar insurance coverage, so we provided it. Whether we would have done differently if we had known what we know today is immaterial. What's done is done."

What's done isn't easily undone, but GM is trying, according to Zink. "Many major employers believe that we would have a better chance of keeping cost increases at a more reasonable level if we could bring about some changes in our coverages," he said, "changes that would create some concern on the part of the patient about costs and communicate this concern effectively to the doctors and hospitals. Practically every new health care benefit introduced into the auto industry over the past 10 years has contained copayment provisions. But we have failed completely in our efforts to get participation by the patient at the point of service in the hospitals—our most expensive coverage. The UAW is strongly opposed. So is the AFL-CIO. Nevertheless, in our next national negotiations with the unions in 1979, we'll try again."

Meanwhile, GM is making its own efforts to communicate its concern effectively to doctors and hospitals, Zink reported. "We have asked our people to become involved in the health care system where they work and live," he said. "For example, we have asked them to become active, questioning members of hospital boards, not to check their brains with their hats at the door of the board room. We have the seminars with knowledge-able faculty to help our involved management personnel under-stand the issues and take a more active part in what is done on behalf of their hospitals and their communities." In these sessions, Zink said, trustees were told to get their hospitals to establish cost containment committees appointed by the boards, think of their total communities, not just their own institutions, create chances to shrink the system, and in capital investment decisions to ask, "What would really happen if we didn't make this investment?" The trustees were also urged to keep abreast of community data on occupancy levels, length of stay, utilization, and number of employees per patient and to "start asking searching questions and don't stop until you get reasonable answers." General Motors now has more than 150 people actively devoting time and attention to hospitals, local health planning agencies, and Blue Cross-Blue Shield boards, Zink reported. "It's not an easy way to go," he concluded. "Some of our people are actually at loggerheads with each other. In one location, for example, one of our engineers who is president of a hospital board is suing the local HSA, the chairman of which is on our financial staff. But this is just an indication of how difficult it is. We hope we can help all of them to do a better job."

General Motors isn't out there all by itself. At Alcoa, where health care costs last year came to 71 percent of net income, corporate policy includes pushing HMOs and encouraging employees to serve on HSA and hospital boards, and a survey of 16 communities having Alcoa plants discovered 19 Alcoans on hospital boards, four of them as presidents. "At one West Coast location the manager of our plant was the key to consolidation of two community hospitals," said an Alcoa report. "At another location in the Midwest the manager of our facility has been working for over five years to accomplish a merger of two community hospitals, as chairman of a task force which undertook the study of consolidation. The activities of our manager and other industrial and civic leaders resulted in articles of incorporation approved by both boards."

Back in 1972, when Motorola was exchanging brickbats with hospitals in Arizona, an executive of the Goodyear Tire and

Rubber Company was worrying about an errant statistic: The average length of hospital stay for Goodyear employees in Akron was two days higher than the national average. This was of direct concern to Richard Martin, Goodyear's manager of health service industry relations, because Goodyear is self-insured; instead of buying health insurance for its employees, Goodyear simply pays their bills, and Martin thought the bills were higher than they should be. To find out why, and what could be done about it, Martin arranged to have the Medical Advances Institute (MAI), Ohio's PSRO Support Center, conduct concurrent review of the care of Goodyear patients at Akron City Hospital. As it turned out, the review pinpointed the problem, and MAI data made it possible for the medical staff to initiate corrective measures. Later, Martin helped get review programs started at hospitals in communities where Goodyear has plants. But "Goodyear isn' t doing this. I don't think we should be in the business of medical audits. Let the doctors do that."

Like General Motors, Goodyear believes in attacking health care costs from all sides. In Akron, Martin is president of the Summit-Portage County HSA, and other company managers are involved in HSA board and committee activities—a circumstance that may have something to do with the agency's three-year record of turning down a larger volume of hospital projects than it approved. "There is almost no limit to what you can do in the HSA if you begin drawing on your company resources," Martin told a conference on industry's role in health care. Financial people, industrial relations people, construction people, and others from industry can all make contributions, he suggested."The potential for hospitals to achieve savings in all these areas is substantial," he said. But there isn't any one approach that will work for all areas, Martin believes. "In some places we're looking at HMOs, or second surgical opinions, or helping hospitals with their voluntary cost containment efforts," he told a reporter recently. "What we're trying to do is help improve the whole system, not just parts of it."

Improving the whole system is also the big idea of the Washington Business Group on Health (WBGH), which was organized under the leadership of Charles J. Pilliod Jr., Goodyear's board chairman, who was chairman of the health task force of the Business Roundtable. WBGH started with five companies and has grown in a few years to include 150 members providing health care benefits for more than 30 million employees, retirees, and dependents. In a monograph published earlier this year, Willis B. Goldbeck, WBGH executive director, explained the organization's purpose. "Although unabashedly desirous of influencing the future direction of health policy, industry needed a vehicle for involvement that differentiated itself from traditional corporate lobbying organizations and tactics," he said. "The theory was, and is, that if the industry resource is valid, its presence will be felt through substantive work that could not be limited to the headline issues like national health insurance. To gain the level of respect necessary to have an impact on these issues, the industry resource had to be applied to many immediate and, by comparison, smaller health care issues."[1]

Gathering, analyzing, and disseminating information furnished by its member companies, WBGH has studied smaller issues such as reimbursement of providers, planning, health insurance practice, HMOs, and health education, and Goldbeck has policy recommendations for industry participation, along with government and providers, in all these activities. "Industry can be the agent for change," he said. "It has the financial resources and the financial incentives. It is just awakening to the realization of its potential. Industry should not be given the responsibility for directing change. Rather, it should take the responsibiltiy for assisting in orderly progress."

From a source providing health care benefits for 30 million people, this would appear to be a reasonable, and even modest, expectation, but it makes some providers nervous to have industry, as well as government, peering over their shoulders. "You admit that your own insurance coverage is responsible for a large share of the cost increase," an administrator told Zink at the financial managers' meeting, "but now you want us to make all the changes to hold costs down." At another conference, a physician took exception to the report that corporations are urging their executives to serve on hospital boards and telling them how to act. "The whole idea seems to be to cut costs," he said. "What is that going to do to patient care? I don't want trustees selected that way on the board of the hospital where I take my patients!"

It is possible to sympathize with these views without agreeing with them. Physicians and hospital administrators are understandably sensitive at a time of unprecedented harassment of the health care establishment, but the questions industry's programs for hospital trustees are teaching them to ask are the questions trustees should have been asking right along, and there isn't any evidence that industry's concern for cost is going to be harder on patient care than government's or, for that matter, the voluntary cost containment effort's is. It may be, in fact, that the industry influence will help protect hospitals from the rudest harassment of all. "We cannot support direct price controls," WBGH said in a working paper sent to HEW Secretary Joseph Califano last year. "We take that position not only because we are philosophically opposed, but also because there is ample evidence that such programs do not work, no matter how carefully designed."

The issue, at any rate, isn't simply to spend less, but to spend less unproductively, and, as Goldbeck has pointed out, that could mean some form of rationing. "This is an emotionally charged issue, all the more difficult in an era of affluence and the public perception that medical care has become a right for all," he said. "Rationing, however, is not new. It has occurred and does occur on all levels. When Congress funds an institute for one disease rather than another, that is rationing. The same can be said of administration policy. The major new emphasis on child health programs means there will not be a major new emphasis on some other worthy population category or research item. Similar rationing is conducted by employers and unions when they negotiate to provide insurance for heart surgery but not for psychiatric care. Providers ration care for us as they select among alternative treatment modalities, or by their refusal, rare but far from nonexistent, to treat without prior evidence of ability to pay, or even by the allocation of scarce funds for one type of machine over another. It is time we stopped fearing the concept of rationing and began to face its reality. In the years ahead, limited resources, expanding expectations, new medical technology, and rising costs will inevitably force us to make even harder decisions. The only alternative to the eventual allocation of all medical and health care resources by government is an immediate and continuous improvement in our utilization of the resources now available."

Meanwhile, it is an illuminating phenomenon of industry's

commitment to the big idea of health that many if not most of the WBGH companies, and hundreds of others, are actively engaged in providing preventive services, health education, and fitness programs for employees, all aimed at doing something, instead of just talking, about the need to motivate people to take more responsibility for their own health, and teaching them how. In all these new directions of concern about health, it is interesting to observe that the professions, presumably guided by an ethic that says do what's right, not what pays, hang back and ask, Is it cost effective? How do we know? Where are the data?—while industry, supposedly hard-nosed and profit-minded, accepts the proposition as a matter of conviction and acts without waiting around for the data. There must be a lesson here somewhere, but maybe we'd rather not know what it is.

[1]Goldbeck, Willis B., A Business Perspective on Industry and Health Care. Springer Series on Industry and Health Care, Number 2, New York: Springer-Verlag New York, Inc., 1978.

Give Us Goals,
But Not Methods

September 1978

According to a recent opinion poll, 70 percent of the American people think the health care system is out of control and needs to be changed, even though 86 percent of those who had been hospitalized said they were satisfied with their care. This apparent contradiction, which has been noted repeatedly in the polls and varies only according to the way the questions are asked, can probably be explained by the fact that lawmakers and government officials at all levels, insurance executives, employers, union leaders, and consumer organizers are all in a panic about the amounts that are being spent on health services for the groups they represent. They all make pronouncements on the subject, and what they say is reported every day in newspaper headlines and columns and by television reporters and commentators. So when an opinion poll interviewer asks a respondent if he thinks the health care system is out of control and needs to be changed, of course he is going to be disposed to say yes, because any other answer would be equivalent to saying, "I am an idiot who doesn't know what is going on in the world."

This "idiot effect" was also apparent when opinions about cost containment measures were examined. Details of the cost containment sections of the report suggested that most people would like to see "inflation in health care costs reduced," as the proposition was stated, by measures like preadmission tests, second surgical opinions, outpatient surgery, and "making hospital patients pay the first small part of their bills," in the delicate phraseology of opinion polls. But there was a strong feeling that cost controls shouldn't be imposed by government. As one of the nation's leading opinion research practitioners summed it up, "Despite the public's complaints about hospital costs and support for some cost-containing measures, the Amer-

103

ican public wants the best available care and is willing to pay for it."[1] That much we already knew.

If this is actually the case, if public concern is only a reflection, and not the cause, of the concern of public officials, and if people really want the best care and are willing to pay for it, why do we need regulation?

Of course, it's a lot more complicated than that. Obviously, the answers are many and complex, and they lie deeply buried in the imperfections not just of the health care system but of the political system, which was planned to provide for the management of public affairs by the most knowledgeable and thoughtful and selfless citizens who could be found, but it hasn't turned out exactly that way. Similarly, the freedoms and privileges society has accorded the health professions are based on the underlying assumption that their behavior will be guided by the ethic that places service to mankind ahead of gain and preferment for themselves, and it hasn't always worked out that way, either. And a third set of complexities arises from the fact that the effectiveness of all our social and political institutions depends on a degree of fair and reasonable use by a populace that is often unfair and unreasonable. Given elected and appointed public officials for whom reelection and reappointment may at any time take precedence over the public interest, physicians and health care administrators motivated as much on occasion by profit and aggrandizement as by the needs of their patients and communities, and a population that can be either generous or greedy or bright or dumb or wise or foolish, and is often all these at once, what can we expect the health care system to look like?

Probably it couldn't look any different from the way it does, which depends on who's looking. Those who would like to see government with a lesser role think it's already socialistic, those who want government to take a stronger hand call it obese, or worse, and those who like the way it looks, or at least are not too disaffected, call it pluralistic, which may mean only that the things they don't want to do should be somebody else's job. Those who never give it a thought until they get sick, when they want care right away at any cost, are likely to call it whatever an interviewer may suggest, such as "out of control and needing change."

These divergent and often contradictory views of what the

health care system is and what it should be make it unlikely that there will be any early resolution of the tangled confusion of regulation that has emerged in the effort to compensate for so many imperfections in human beings and the systems they try to create and manage. It is an article of faith among hardline individualists in the health professions that the National Health Planning and Resources Development Act of 1974 and the regulations that followed on its enactment, for example, are at the core of a far-reaching government plan to seize control of the entire health care apparatus, and it is equally an article of faith among some of the visionaries in the Congress and the bureaus that the health professions and institutions have no end in view save their own advantage and would evade or thwart the purposes of the planning act if they couldn't abolish it altogether. This kind of worry about intentions is witless; we don't by any means always understand our own intentions, much less anybody else's. It seems more sensible to believe that all either side really wants is a health care system that works without giving away the store, on the one hand, or overcharging the customers on the other.

The planning act itself calls for priority consideration of the provision of primary care services for medically underserved populations, the development of medical group practices appropriately coordinated or integrated with institutional health services, increased utilization of physicians' assistants, multi-institutional arrangements for the sharing of support services, development of the capacity to provide various levels of care on a geographically integrated basis, promotion of activities for the prevention of disease, adoption of uniform cost accounting, simplified reimbursement, and utilization reporting systems, and development of effective methods of educating the public concerning proper personal health care and effective use of available services. It is barely possible to read this list of national health priorities as a blueprint to remodel the premises, but it is also possible to believe instead that the objective is simply to remedy what are some of the more visible gaps and flaws in the system—granted that those who are well served and well pleased with what we have now are something less than wildly enthusiastic about some of these goals.

The planning guidelines may be something else. As they were first proposed last November, for those with lifetime commitments to existing practices and institutions the guidelines had all the impact of a call to revolution. As best, they were a heavy-footed attempt to leap from where we are now to where some of the less informed and more inflamed among the functionaries of government thought we ought to be. As the guidelines emerged eventually after the initial uproar subsided, the call to revolution was muted but not wholly silenced, and it seems likely now that with further modification and sensible application in the provinces, where the trumpets of the Czar may be heard but are not always heeded, the system can survive the battle of the guidelines.

As it is working out in practice after four years, the planning act and its regulatory appurtenances haven't made all that much difference in the way people behave; jumping through the required hoops takes time and costs money, but up to now it hasn't changed where anybody stands. There have been some monumental miscarriages of good sense, to be sure. In Massachusetts, for example, errors of interpretation and judgment on the part of poorly informed bureaucrats have so harassed and hampered such exceptional and needed institutions as the world-renowned Lahey Clinic and the Tufts-New England Medical Center as to seriously impair their usefulness, if not their excellence. And in Oklahoma the combined efforts of the health professions and the planners, on the same side for once, were unable to prevent the state's political apparatus from approving construction of an unneeded and fantastically expensive medical center for Oral Roberts University in Tulsa, where just about everybody acknowledges there are too many beds already. The ostensible reason for this aberration was that the new medical center would become a world-wide referral center for millions of believers in the Oral Roberts faith; the real reason was statehouse clout. In Tulsa, it isn't the health care system that is out of control and needs change. It's the political system.

For every Oral Roberts, however, there are HSAs and state planning boards negotiating change with physicians and institutions, not easily or painlessly but without seriously disrupting the existing system or vitiating the purposes of the act, and for every Lahey Clinic there is a professional health care community coping with its planners and politicians and either meeting or modifying their requirements and staying in business—as in fact, for all its expensive delays and detours, the Lahey Clinic has done. On the evidence to date, the doomsayers who saw the National Health Planning and Resources Development Act as the end of the voluntary health care system were wrong. If the end should come in our time, the cause is more likely to be some combination of inadequate reimbursement, inflation, and depression, not planning or regulation *per se*.

Contemplating the impenetrable thicket of laws and rules surrounding their operations, hospital administrators and physicians often get the idea that the health care system has been singled out for oppressive restraints, while the rest of the society goes its carefree, uninhibited way. But as hospital trustees in the utilities, banking, transportation, petroleum, and other heavily regulated industries know, that isn't the case at all, and indeed few if any of us are entirely free of the regulatory web. In what may be the closest parallel to the hospital predicament, school boards and administrators are facing declining pupil populations, diminishing state aid, dissatisfied teachers, demanding unions, and multiplying state and federal regulations governing finance, jurisdiction, racial integration, and, increasingly, educational programming. To one degree or another, corporate boards of directors and executives are caught up in the same plexus of rules, not because anybody in the government wants to nationalize the economy but because rules governing corporate behavior have become essential in an industrial society, for the same reasons rules governing the behavior of health care professions and institutions are necessary. A thoughtful industrialist who is as familiar with the constraints of regulations as any hospital administrator could be made the reasons clear. "I believe that industry, and I include the energy industry, needs an appropriate measure of regulation," Jerry McAfee, chairman of the board and chief executive officer of the Gulf Oil Corporation, said. "By this I mean that the people of the nation, through their government, should set the bounds within which they want industry to operate. But the rules have got to be clear. Society must spell out clearly what it is it wants the corporations to do. Making the rules straight and understandable is really what government is all about. Set the goals, set the fences, set the criteria, set the atmosphere, but don't tell us how to do it. Tell us what you want made, but don't tell us how to make it. Tell us the destination we're seeking, but don't tell us how to get there."[2]

In health care, some of the rules are not what anybody would call clear and precise, and some of them go beyond goals and boundaries to methods, and this is where most of the pain is felt. It isn't likely that either industry or the health care system will achieve the kind of balanced relationship with government envisioned by McAfee—not soon, certainly. But it isn't impossible, either, and it is certain that we can come closer to it in health care than we have come so far. The making of laws and rules governing health care professions and institutions is still new. The lawmakers and rulemakers are still learning the territory; if they can be helped by the professions and institutions to reach more settled conclusions about the goals, the fences, the criteria, and the atmosphere, it should be possible eventually to resolve the confusion about methods. But we'll never get anywhere mistrusting intentions.

[1]Harris, Louis, quoted in a news release from Hospital Affiliates International, Inc., Health Care in America, the complete survey report can be obtained from Hospital Affiliates International, Inc., free of charge.

[2]McAfee, J., How Society Can Help Business, Newsweek, July 3, 1978, p. 15.

The HMOs Are Coming—
Or Are They?

June 1979

A few weeks ago I had occasion to talk to a group that included representatives of medicine and hospitals, government, universities, health insurance, industry, and labor. The subject of their conference was health care in the American economy, and I had been invited, as sometimes happens, to present the views of a reporter, someone who doesn't represent anyone or manage anything and whose perspective is therefore presumed to be free of bias—an expedient that is clouded, in the opinion of some, by the countervailing circumstance that he doesn't really know anything, either. This last is not an opinion that I share, but it is often called to my attention, at times with a certain amount of vigor.

This was one such time. Among other things, I had commented on the current resurgence of interest in prepaid group practice, or in the contemporary vernacular, HMOs, an arrangement whose economic logic is attractive but whose popularity rises and falls like the ocean tides, and, like the tides, seems always to reach about the same stage, and then recede. HMOs enjoy the high regard of government officials, members of Congress, consultants, professors, economists, business executives, and pundits, I suggested, and are commonly seen by all these and others as the "alternative delivery system" that offers the best answer to the perplexing problems of ever mounting cost. "Everybody loves HMOs," I said, "except for two groups. The two groups are doctors and patients. Doctors don't want to practice that way, and patients don't know what you're talking about."

After the meeting, just two persons had something to say about my reporter's observations. One was an old friend who is on the staff of a well-established and well-known HMO. "You're wrong, you know," he said. "Doctors love HMOs. It's only the

109 "}

patients that are holding back." The other comment came from a health care public relations consultant. "You're wrong, you know," he said. "Patients love HMOs. It's the doctors that are holding back."

Somebody is. Considering the number and stature of the federal officials, lawmakers, economists, business leaders, and others who have been beating the HMO drums, one would think we might have 2,000 HMOs by this time instead of 200, with 70 million members instead of seven million. The number is growing, to be sure, and the rate of growth has been picking up with the introduction of Individual Practice Associations. The IPA is a kind of back-door HMO that offers comprehensive service at fixed annual rates but allows its doctors to keep their private practice and pays them on a fee-for-service basis, thus diminishing resistance by doctors and improving accessibility for subscribers, but limiting the cost saving that is seen as the principal advantage of the HMO. In the Twin Cities area of Minneapolis-St. Paul, for example, where there are seven HMO-type plans now in operation, the average utilization rate for all the HMOs is 548 hospital days per 1,000 population per year, compared with 720 days for Blue Cross-Blue Shield and private insurance patients, according to a report from the Minnesota State Department of Health. The utilization of the one IPA plan in the area is 639 days, so the saving in days is about half that of the HMOs. With so many HMOs and correspondingly large numbers of physicians and subscribers, the Twin Cities area is considered a showcase of HMO progress outside of Kaiser territory, so it is a measure of the state of the art that total HMO-IPA enrollment is estimated at 255,000—about 12 percent of the area's population and less than a third the number enrolled in Blue Cross and Blue Shield groups.

Asked how it is that HMOs can have so many priests and so few converts still, the movement's missionaries commonly reply that the idea is new, and it takes time for any new approach to gain acceptance among doctors and patients. But the HMO idea really isn't new all all. The basic element, physician acceptance of responsibility for care of defined populations, usually at a fixed price paid in advance, has been around in one form or another ever since the days of the sick clubs and friendly societies of Europe in the Middle Ages. In this country, George Washington and his fellow plantation owners paid physicians to take care of their slaves, and much the same arrangement prevailed in the 19th and early 20th centuries in company towns of the railroad, mining, and lumber industries, where the corporations paid the doctors and often collected from the workers, who were not known as slaves.

Then in 1937, at a time when "group hospitalization," as it was called, was catching on in a few large cities and was just beginning to be known as Blue Cross, an HMO that had been organized by employees of the Home Owners' Loan Corp. in Washington, DC, the Group Health Association, Inc., was a cause of controversy among Washington physicians. The District of Columbia Medical Society had asked the American Medical Association for help in "meeting the threat of that organization,"[1] and a year later a special grand jury was appointed to investigate charges by U.S. assistant attorney general Thurman Arnold that the AMA and the district society had conspired to limit the freedom of Group Health physicians by denying them access to hospital facilities. The grand jury returned indictments, and following a U.S. court of appeals decision reversing an earlier ruling that medicine was not a trade within the scope of the Sherman Antitrust Act, the case went to trial in 1940 before a jury that included businessmen, housewives, and one federal employee.

The trial went on for months and concluded finally with an evenhanded charge to the jury by U.S. district court justice James M. Proctor: "The defendants have the right to adopt rules for just and fair dealing among their members and a right of enforcement of those rules and regulations by such reasonable penalties as they may provide for violation thereof," the court said in part, referring to the medical societies and 21 of their officers named in the indictments. "The defendants had the right to reach and attempt to reach their objective of advancing the interests of the medical profession by legitimate persuasion and reasoned argument, and to this end they had the right to tell their side of the story and to persuade others, including the Washington hospitals, other physicians, members of Group Health Association, Inc., and the public to utilize and use the defendants' method of practicing medicine, and to use peaceful persuasion, publicity, articles in the press, in publications of defendants, including the *Journal of the American Medical Association*, and all lawful propaganda to have their methods of practicing medicine prevail over those of Group Health Association.

"The hospitals had the lawful right to prescribe rules and regulations governing the use of their facilities by doctors and patients. In their boards was vested the authority to decide what physicians would be allowed the privileges. A doctor had no right to demand them. To grant or refuse the same rested solely with the hospital. Therefore, if denial of privileges to members of the Group Health staff represented the voluntary decision of the boards, no question would arise as to the legality of their acts. However, if refusal was arbitrary and to serve a criminal conspiracy against Group Health or their doctors, it would violate the statute. The respective merits of different methods of medical care are not an issue in this case. Advocates and adherents of each are entitled to their views and may follow their choice. They had the right to support the same by fair competition and to oppose by way of discussion, argument, and persuasion. But neither group would be justified in conspiring to restrain the activities of the other . . . If you find that the defendants conspired together for the purposes charged, and if you find that the defendants, in seeking to achieve those purposes, intended to prevent Group Health Association physicians from competing with doctors engaged in private practice on a fee-for-service basis in furnishing medical care to members of the public eligible for membership in Group Health Association, then the defendants were engaged in a combination in restraint of trade."[2]

In a curious verdict, the jury decided that the AMA and the District of Columbia Medical Society were guilty of the conspiracy charge, but all the defendant officers of both organizations were innocent. The logic of the decision escapes comprehension, but there isn't much question that the trial, if not the verdict, had a dampening effect on the growth of prepaid group practice that persisted for years but has largely vanished in our time as various professional groups, including the AMA, have joined government agencies, business organizations, and others in voicing approval of the concept—on occasion with restrained enthusiasm.

Without exception, the committees and commissions that have studied the subject lean heavily in their reports and recommendations on the experience of the modern prototype HMO, the Kaiser Foundation Health Plan and Permanente

Medical Groups. Kaiser's history began at Grand Coulee Dam in the state of Washington in 1938 when Henry and Edgar Kaiser, father and son, invited Sidney R. Garfield, M.D., to come form a medical group to provide care for 10,000 dam workers and their families, something Garfield had already done for a smaller group of aqueduct workers in southern California, beginning in 1933. The plans worked, and the Kaisers transplanted them and Garfield to their shipyards and steel mills in California, Oregon, and Washington during World War II. When the plans were opened to the public after the war, however, physician recruitment became a problem because organized medicine for the most part was still convinced that closed-panel practice lowered the quality of medical care and threatened the citadels of private practice. Permanente Group doctors continued to have a hard time in some Kaiser communities until 1959, when the report of an AMA Commission on Medical Care headed by Leonard Larson, M.D., said its investigations found the quality of care in prepaid group practice equal to the quality in fee-for-service practice, and better in some low-income areas where care was hard to get.

The Larson report was the end of the line of organized medical opposition to prepaid group practice, but that doesn't mean doctors everywhere have changed the way they feel about it. Some have, but many still regard it as somehow professionally inferior, and in some communities this attitude has been reinforced as groups lacking adequate knowledge, experience, sponsorship, funds, or management skills have sought to start HMOs, sometimes with the good intention of making comprehensive care more readily accessible where a need has appeared, but sometimes, unfortunately, with the desire only to make money by offering an attractive-looking package to underserved Medicaid populations. It seems most likely, however, that the great majority of practicing physicians are neither for nor against HMOs per se but are simply satisfied with their own practices and see no reason to change. For such physicians, the inclination to resist changes may owe something to the governmental and professional zealots whose HMO hosannas declare or imply that private practice is either inefficient or avaricious or both. Whatever they are, the causes for physician resistance seem to be softened in the case of the IPA model—but so are the causes for hosannas.

As well as it can be done, recent public opinion polls probably tell the reason Americans haven't been knocking down the doors of HMOs to sign up as soon as they are in business: Eighty-percent or more of people queried say they are satisfied with the medical care they are getting now, and despite the shrieking headlines and lamentations about cost, in one of the polls that asked specifically about dissatisfactions, only 37 percent named cost as the principal reason—a circumstance that has to mean 63 percent were not that dissatisfied even with the cost. Whenever this seeming public indifference to the cost of medical care is mentioned, government officials and others who like to envision an outraged citizenry marching on hospitals are quick to point out that it is the insurance system that keeps people from knowing how much their care is costing. This is unquestionably true, to some extent, and certainly the public concern about cost would be greater if patients were paying a larger share of the bill at the time medical services are required. But knowing this is the case doesn't really solve anything, because employers are not likely to go back now and take away the relatively unrestricted benefits employees and their unions have bargained for and enjoyed for years.

In any event, the competition or the choice of alternative systems so many reformers advocate so passionately doesn't seem to work as well as they think it should. After 40 years, Kaiser covers something less than 15 percent of the population of the West Coast states that are considered Kaiser country, and its carefully planned and marketed forays into Colorado and Ohio have not exactly swept those populations off their feet. But the Colorado and Ohio plans are stable and growing, and this month Kaiser and the Prudential Insurance Co. expect to commence operation of an HMO that has been in development for two years in the Dallas-Fort Worth area. Better than most if not all others, Kaiser knows how. "It is not easy to do," a Kaiser official told a reporter who made an extensive study for the Kaiser Foundation a few years ago. "If anyone asked me to say what is our major problem in one sentence, it would be how to keep our balance—facilities, doctors, paramedical personnel, patients."[3]

Concluding his investigation, the reporter had an explanation for the slow consumer swing to group practice plans. "People are inclined to stick with what they have and assume that what they have is best," he said. "One thing the East has lacked is a Henry J. Kaiser, a maverick industrialist with a driving interest in people's health and, in this direction, no profit motive. He loved doctors and medicine, was afraid of nobody, and was convinced he could make anything happen."

They broke the mold when Henry Kaiser died in 1967, but there are signs that new interest in HMOs is awakening in industry. R.J. Reynolds Industries has started a group practice plan for its employees at Winston-Salem, NC; in an unequaled burst of management-labor-professional brotherly love the automobile industry, the UAW, and the Henry Ford Hospital have joined hands to resurrect the Metro Health Plan, a Detroit HMO that has been going for 20 years; and another group of corporation chairmen and union presidents has been meeting in Washington planning to push HMOs and other health reforms. Among other things, the group has recommended that industry should make capital loans and loan guarantees available to HMOs and provide technical assistance for HMO development and funds for training medical and marketing directors and administrators of HMOs.

All this should help, if anybody is listening, but it still isn't going to be easy, for reasons that were made clear at HEW Secretary Joseph Califano's 1978 HMO pep meeting when a public utilities executive said his company had been offering an HMO option to its employees for 10 years. "The HMO enrollment got up to six percent and leveled off there, with as many dropping out and going back to Blue Cross-Blue Shield as there were joining the HMO," he reported. There must be a reason for this, and there must be a reason an arrangement that has been known since George Washington's time now has a total of seven million members, give or take, while Blue Cross-Blue Shield and insurance have enrolled 180 million Americans in a single generation. Many reasons have been suggested, but it may be that the simplest reason is nearest to the truth: That's the way the doctors and the people want it, and they are the only ones who can really determine what happens. Theorists argue that the problem in health care is the absence of market forces and propose more regulation to correct what they see as imbalance, but HMO history suggests that where the market does exist, the choice has been mostly against prepaid group practice. Defenders of the HMO faith point out that these have not been fair competitive tests, because of tax advantages offered employers and employees under Internal Revenue Service rulings on existing health insurance, and because in most markets there aren't enough HMO or IPA alternatives to offer realistic choices. As evidence, they point to Minneapolis-St. Paul and areas in California where the percentage of total population enrolled in HMOs may remain low, but where employers do offer a real multiple choice of health care plans and as many as 20 or 30 percent or more are choosing an alternative to traditional fee-for-service coverage. When this happens, they say, doctors can't afford to remain indifferent and hospitals have to compete for the HMO business, and market forces operate to hold costs down.

With industry and government and some union and consumer groups all pushing, the swing to HMOs that only the missionaries have seen so far could materialize in time, but even the enthusiasts acknowledge that the pace will be stately. At whatever size and speed, however, the swing should be welcomed as an antidote to a disease that was identified by a New York physician and that he said was threatening to become endemic in the health care system. He called it hardening of the categories.

[1]Fishbein, M., A History of the American Medical Association 1847 to 1947, Philadelphia: W.B. Saunders Co., 1947, pp. 430-32.

[2]ibid., pp. 547-50.

[3]Williams, G., Kaiser Plan: The Prepaid Group Practice Model and How It Grew, Modern Hospital, 116:2, February 1971.

The Voluntary Spirit Is Alive and Well

September 1980

Just a few years ago, it was a popular indoor sport among critics of the health services in the United States to protest whenever we referred to the health care system and object scornfully that it wasn't really a system at all. When they were in good form, the critics delighted in calling it a nonsystem, obviously intending that to mean that it couldn't be worse. This particular criticism hasn't been heard so much in the past two or three years, not because the critics consider that there has been any notable progress toward making a system out of what they had seen as a nonsystem, but mainly because changing economic and political circumstance has focused their whole attention on another problem: Whatever it is, it costs too much and ought to be changed. There is no agreement among the critics on what it ought to be changed to, as long as it costs less.

If we are to consider that a system is an aggregation of diverse parts so organized as to provide unity or coherence contributing to some common purpose shared by the parts, which is what most of us mean when we use the word thoughtfully, then it is fair to say that we probably don't have a health care system in the United States today, or at best we have a system that is imperfectly organized and lacking in coherence. What we have instead is a multiplicity of systems—separate systems for the military services, and another system for veterans; a separate system for people over age 65, and another for disadvantaged mothers and infants, and still another for the poor and near poor. Some of the systems are complete and coherent and provide a full range of services for their assigned populations. Others, like Medicare and Medicaid, are financing systems, or partial financing systems, whose populations depend for the entitled services on still other systems, loosely so called, such as physicians in private practice by themselves or in groups; indi-

117

vidual hospitals or hospital systems organized in a variety of ways, as by ownership or region; nursing homes of even greater diversity; health maintenance organizations of all sizes and types. The same systems of institutional and professional services provide care for that segment of the population not included in any of the public financing systems but in private financing systems such as Blue Cross and Blue Shield Plans, insurance companies, HMOs, and payment systems organized by employers, unions, fraternal groups, and others.

Given the number and diffusion of our health care systems, the remarkable thing is not that the whole aggregation has been referred to as a nonsystem by only a small number of the crankier critics, while the rest of us keep on thinking of it, and calling it, a system as though it were a coherent, organized unity of some kind. The remarkable thing is not that it works imperfectly, but that it works at all and doesn't fly apart, and it may be instructive to consider the reasons it doesn't. For one thing, it is only recently, since the cost flap started, that anybody except the critics cared whether it was a system or not. We called it that unthinkingly, the same way everybody was calling everything a system after the word emerged from the war and space technology and was picked up by Madison Avenue and the business schools and all the salesmen started pushing cleaning systems instead of carpet sweepers and photographic systems instead of cameras. Another reason is that while we do have all these separate, diverse, diffused parts, and they do overlap in some places and leave gaps in others and aren't very well integrated anywhere, the whole thing doesn't work all that badly. In fact, for most of us it works pretty well, and while we certainly need to be doing something more about those who get stuck in the cracks between the parts, the only reason anybody wants even to consider the kind of change that would be required to pull all the parts together into a single system is that the way things are, nobody can get a handle on the cost problem, and nobody is willing to acknowledge that there isn't any handle. So we wring our hands and comfort ourselves with vague talk about system reform, which doesn't mean much of anything except to a few fanatics in the Federal Trade Commission and the Congress and the universities who are obsessed with the idea that what we need to solve all the problems of the health services is price competition among doctors and hospitals, and to them "system reform" is code, meaning "push HMOs."

Obviously, there is some exaggeration in the description here of the diversity of our health care systems, because except for the closed military and veterans systems, and to some extent the mental and public hospital systems, the majority of the population, whatever the methods of financing their care, are served by the private practice and voluntary hospital systems, and while there is about as much diversity within these systems as anybody can stand, at the same time there is enough commonality of form and purpose among the parts to make it permissible to refer to the whole thing as a system, if anybody wants to and thinks it is important to do. And in spite of the inroads on independence of the units in the era of public entitlements introduced by Medicare and Medicaid, there is enough freedom of action and decision here still to make it permissible to call it a voluntary system, and this is an important qualifier.

Will it stay like this? Will the voluntary principle survive? The only sensible answer is that depends, and it depends on a lot of things. For example, if our friendly leaders and those who are running around the country trying to remain or become our friendly leaders get completely carried away and get us into another war, voluntarism will vanish not only from our health care system but probably from our lives as well. If the unmanageable inflation continues to push prices out of sight, including health care prices, it seems certain to bring on the kind of control measures that would take another bite out of the voluntary principle. And even if the inflation should get all the way back to where we can live with it, some economists are coming to the view that we are not likely soon, if ever, to return to the kind of economic growth that kept inflation and unemployment at arm's length for 30 years.

But along with the gloomy outlook for economic growth, and the aging population, and the continued inflation, and the putative or probable failure of competitive therapy, and the increasing regulation, and the erosion of voluntarism, there are one or two countervailing forces that have to be considered too. These are not likely to reverse the course of events and take us back to a time when the principal preoccupation of hospital executives and trustees was whether to increase the room rate first and then the service charges or do it the other way around, and in any case whether to do it now or wait until the new addition is completed and occupied. Whether we are talking about the whole system or any of its parts or institutions, the job is going to be one of allocating limited resources—deciding what or whom to leave out, or rationing care.

One of the countervailing forces that could delay the onset or curb the severity of any further invasions of voluntarism might be the ongoing technology, which some of the optimists among the economic oracles think may yet resolve the energy crisis and relieve the inflation. In health care, the principal effect of technologic advance over the past generation has been to prolong life and add expense, but it is possible, at least, that some future technology may ease the burden on the health care system without notably adding to its problems. About the only thing that can be said with certainty about the technology is that it isn't going to be turned off by any evaluation or assessment procedures laid on by planning regulation, though these measures may from time to time divert the deployment of new technology, as has already happened. But technology assessment, like regional planning, is likely to continue colliding head-on all over the place with another of the countervailing forces—one that is a lot more solidly established in our culture than either regional planning or technology assessment—local pride, local autonomy, and local initiative. In this as in most human affairs, you win some and you lose some, but up to now local initiative has won more than it has lost in the collisions with regional planning and technology assessment. The balance of power could shift over time, but it will never be a runaway.

Local initiative is also at the core of another countervailing force that has been around for a few thousand years. Philanthropy in our time has been losing ground to tax reform, welfarism, and inflation, and the role of philanthropy in health care has been diminished further with the advent of Medicare and Medicaid and the increasing tendency of hospitals to be regarded more as, and act more like, businesses. But a human trait that has been practiced in every known civilization, and honored in every known religion, is not about to disappear, and, in fact, there is evidence that hospitals are taking a renewed interest in philanthropy as regulatory authority tightens its grip on patient revenues. Philanthropy is a long way from being counted out, and as long as philanthropy is alive, the voluntary principle lives.

Finally, there is the new interest in wellness. Nobody really knows yet whether or not it will pay off for industry, but a number of large corporations have been willing to bet that it will and have invested in fitness facilities and programs as well as screening and counseling services and health education activities. Along with the creative power of the technology, local initiative, revived philanthropy, and the probable infusion of some elements of price competition in the health care economy, the wellness movement in industry and in the population at large has to be counted among the forces demonstrating that the voluntary spirit is going to be around for another generation, at least, and as long as the voluntary spirit lasts, the nation's doctors and hospitals will not be found in a health care system whose coherence is laid on from outside.

Competition and Regulation: We Need Them Both

October 1980

When the Congress demonstrates a lot of interest in a subject or a particular piece or type of legislation in a year divisible by four, you can always be sure the position and the vote, if it comes to that, are going to be taken not so much because of the merits of the subject or the principles involved, but because the position and the vote are figured to make the Senators and Congressmen look good back home. This is a commonplace observation, to be sure, as well known to schoolchildren as it is to seasoned lobbyists. But what is known only to lobbyists, and not even to all of them, is that when the position favoring the legislation is simplistic and the position opposing it is complex and abstruse, the opposition is not just "in trouble," as we say. The opposition is going to lose. And the sad part is that it doesn't have to be that way. The voters—the people—are not that dumb. They can take an abstruse issue apart and see what's inside as easily as the politicians and their think-tank advisers and the geniuses of the TV evening news can, but they never get the chance. The assumption is that only the simplistic position will be understood, so even the opposition avoids the complexity and says "Yes, but" instead of "No."

This is the case, in October of this divisible year, with the position and the bills having to do with price competition in the provision of health care services. From Schweiker to Durenberger to Gephardt, the bills are known, and invariably referred to, as *pro*-competition bills. Why *pro*? We didn't refer to the national health insurance bills as *pro*-NHI. We didn't call the National Health Planning and Resources Development Act the *pro*-planning Act. We don't call tax bills *pro*-tax, or safety bills *pro*-safety, or defense bills *pro*-defense. So why *pro*-competition?

The reason for the label is obvious and important and precisely defines the problem and explains the likelihood that one of the present bills, or a derivative that is even more screwed up than the original, will become law. The reason the bills are so labeled and so universally described is that nobody on any side of any of the complex issues involved in anything having to do with health care—nobody in America, in fact, with the possible exception of aging reporters having nothing to lose—can afford to be considered *anti*-competition. The idea of competition is inseparably entwined with the idea of free enterprise, and the whole concept is enshrouded in impenetrable mystique and elevated to the status of theological doctrine. To question the beneficence of competition in the American economy is unthinkable, like biting God. So nobody does. And even though everybody understands that excessive competition produces intractable economic evils, so competition has to be regulated, the pro-competition enthusiasts continue to insist, or pretend, that competition is a substitute for regulation.

Nobody will say so, but the fact is that there hasn't been that much free enterprise around here for generations. The bankers favor competition, but they want the savings and loan people to be regulated, and they are. The dairy industry is for free enterprise, but they want legislation governing the merchandising of oleomargarine, and they got it. The truckers are as competitive as you can get, as long as the taxpayers give them superhighways to tear up, and they do. The publishers hate regulation, but they love the second-class postage privilege and excommunicate anybody who calls it subsidy. The oil companies and utilities are so comfortable with their monopolies that they've forgotten all about the regulation that made them fat. It's all part of the theology, but a lot of it is masquerade.

What we have here is a partly and cautiously competitive capitalist economy, heavily but not altogether unsuccessfully regulated, and it works pretty well for most of the people most of the time. It's in a tailspin right now, especially in the automobile industries, which are suffering from, of all things, competition. But that's *foreign* competition, the bishops of the theological establishment complain. That's different from our good, productive, efficient, domestic competition. And are they preparing to combat this alien competition with good old American free enterprise efficiency—the "free market forces" that are going to work so well in the market for health care services as soon as the Congress gets off its electoral aspects and passes one of the *pro*-competition confections? Well, not exactly. the thing we need here is—uh—regulation. There ought to be a law.

There will be, and its sponsors will declare solemnly in the committees and on the TV panels that the law was needed "to make the industry more competitive," and the people who understand that it was really needed to protect an inefficient industry from the effects of competition will be silent, because you can't be against competition. Not around here. Not even when the Health Care Financing Administration, masquerading in the disguise of competition, goes behind the Congress's back and vitiates the intermediary nomination provision of the Medicare law by replacing an experienced Medicare contractor with another one and then proposing to change the rules so that the new contractor can remain in place, even though complaints about service have risen out of sight.

So it's plain that we are going to have a health care competition law, and, because *de*-regulation is as much a part of the theology as *pro*-competition is, we'll probably get one of the wackier ones, or something like it, that proposes to do away with the planning law, and the PSRO law, and the HMO law, and the Medicare reporting and reimbursement requirements, and all the regulations that go along with these provisions. So nobody will notice that there will be new sets of regulations right away to deal with things like health care areas, and actuarial categories, and qualified health plans, and basic health care services, and a few million other things the new law will instruct the Secretary of Health and Human Services to direct, or authorize, or approve, or decide, or whatever. The more things change....

If it should really turn out to be that crazy, and all these old regulations do disappear, and all the geniuses and assistant geniuses who wrote the bills are sitting around waiting for the competition to drive prices down, you could guess what's going to happen: the damnedest hospital building boom since Aesculapius built his temples of healing. Something the geniuses apparently don't know is that the excesses, or putative excesses, they've been wringing their hands about for the past half-dozen years—empty beds, overutilization, unnecessary services, the whole litany—are caused by competition, not lack of it, and if all the restraints actually should be lifted, that's the way hospitals and doctors are going to compete again, not by advertising and cutting rates. Because they know something else the geniuses apparently don't know: In health care, people not only want what they think is the best, they demand it and think they're entitled to it and are going to get it, even when they have to pay for it themselves and it costs them a lot more than second best would. They'll take second best anything else for a price, but not second best health care.

But they don't pay for it themselves, the bishops argue, and that's the whole point. Their employers pay for most of it, and employers do care about the cost, and that's what the *pro*-competition flap is all about.

Well, we'll see. Some employers probably do care enough to take on all the hassles that are certain to erupt if their employees do shop around and keep on changing deals and doctors, as the *pro*-competition crowd assumes they're going to do to save a dollar here and a dollar there. But since the proposed law prudently says the employer can't contribute anything less than he has been contributing, the chances are there won't be that much change either way. Believe it or not, bishops, most people like their doctors and don't want to change. And the biggest employers, the ones that pay the most for health care because the benefits have been negotiated over years of collective bargaining, are going to do whatever they can within the law to keep the unions happy. Labor trouble can cost a lot more than health care, and neither the unions nor the managements are throwing hats in air and cheering about reopening all the arguments that have already been settled.

Whichever way it goes, there is a possibility that the health care competition rhubarb could help both sides (the yesses and the yes, buts, that is; there aren't any noes, remember?) penetrate the theological mystique far enough to see something that has been there all along: There is fierce competition among doctors and hospitals and health care systems and health insurers; there always has been and there always will be, just as there has been and will be competition among all sectors in the economy, and all groups in the society, and all peoples in the world. Competitiveness is a built-in quality of the human organism, like the opposable thumb. It is neither good nor bad per se; it is just there. It produces violence as often as it produces excellence, and it is as necessary for us to punish the former as it is for us to reward the latter. The whole body of common law, in fact, can be considered a form of regulation aimed at keeping competitiveness under control. Competition in the economy produces excellence and efficiency, and it also produces barbarity and duplicity; it has produced all these in the health care economy in the past, and it will produce all these in the health care economy in the future, no matter what. So competition has to be regulated in the future, as it has been in the past, and the only thing that should concern us here is whether or not adding price to the competition that is already there could save enough to pay what it will cost to keep the competition clean—that is, to find and curb and punish the predators and cheaters price competition will encourage here, as it does elsewhere in the economy, and keep them from hurting people.

And that's what we ought to be talking about, not "free market forces"—whatever they are, and not the simplistic *either* competition *or* regulation the reformers keep demanding. We've always had both, and we still need both.

How Free Is the Free Market Going to Be?

May 1981

These are times when anybody who isn't a little nervous about how things are going to turn out must know something the rest of us don't know. This has to be true of everybody from the hod carrier to the mathematics professor, but in the whole range of places to earn a living there can't be many that are shot through with as many uncertainties today as what we used to call the hospital field but refer to invariably now as the health care industry—in what is certainly one of the least felicitous of our public relations antics, since it tends to blur the distinction between the healing mission, which has the aura if not always the substance of sanctity, and the ends of commerce, which haven't got much of either. The distinction in all prudence is something we should be flaunting, not flouting, if we want our communities to love us in December as they did in May.

The uncertainties that make us all so nervous are endemic in a society determined to embark on a new course that in the nature of things is partly if not largely uncharted, the reasonable explanation being that the shore we are headed toward can't be as rocky as the shore we are leaving. In the hospital field, as I shall stubbornly insist on calling it, the uncertainties are epidemic. In the necessary and almost universally applauded exercise known in the vulgate as getting the government off our backs, for example, we are obviously going to shrink, first, and then probably abandon, the planning apparatus whose roots reach back to the early voluntary agencies 40 years ago but whose latter-day branches and twigs came to cost more to nourish and support than the fruit they produced was worth, in the opinion of those who are running the orchard. Hosannas for good riddance abound, but in the wakeful nights there are second thoughts. Some planning authority, it is expected, will be surrendered by the extinguished community agencies to the states, and whether that is good or bad depends on what state you have in mind. At their worst, the local agencies at least were local; if we have to leave home to get our shins kicked, the statehouse is not unexceptionally an improvement over the White House.

So there is an uncertainty, and here is another. The agents of change and their enthusiastic cheerleaders are confident that there can be no instant replay, even in the absence of restraining regulation, of the building excesses of the 1950s and 1960s. The money isn't there, they say; interest rates are forbidding, and banks are occupied elsewhere. But then a hospital group executive tells friends that his organization will break ground on five new hospitals as soon as the law allows, and others in their communities and offices are seen blowing the dust off blueprints that have been on shelves for years. Maybe a building boom, or a miniboom, wouldn't be such a bad thing. Some of the building plans contemplate ending up with fewer beds, not more, and in some communities employers and consumers will still be attracted as much by facilities and amenities as they will be by price. But a building boom isn't a way to save money.

A former member of the chorus now playing a strong supporting role in the cast a few weeks ago assured an anxious lawmaker that before any irremediable action is taken a new study will be made to determine once and for all whether or not PSRO saves as much as it costs. That would be either the fourth or fifth study to determine once and for all whether or not PSRO saves as much as it costs, and it can be predicted with confidence that this one will prove that (a) PSRO either saves more than it costs or costs more than it saves, (b) the differences will not be great, and (c) in any case the result will be disputed on the ground that the data were inconclusive. But the fact is that PSRO has been losing its constituency. There is a powerful and persuasive new mode of thought, a new force running in the society and determined to cut government down to manageable size, and the government programs that the new force is going to be most successful in dislodging are those with the least constituencies. PSRO has just about run itself out of constituency; the decline is here, and the fall is in sight.

But wait just a minute. Which way are our communities going to look now to be sure quality and medical necessity safeguards are in place and working? The doctors say just leave it to us, we're doing it anyway, but doctors testifying that their colleagues are doing everything right aren't going to be believed by anybody but their colleagues. The Blues have announced a brave new medical necessity program, carefully developed over months of painstaking work with specialty societies. But not all the Plans and providers march when the bugle is sounded, and employers, especially, want actual savings now, not putative savings later. PSRO is expensive, and slow, and often cumbersome, and sometimes infuriating. But it is there, and working, and some companies already are paying PSROs for review of employees' care. Others may do likewise and keep some PSROs in business as government funding is phased out over the coming year, and it is also expected that "competing systems of care" in the envisioned new world will contract for review by surviving PSROs. The dream beats the real thing every time. Meanwhile, if Medicare and Medicaid are still around and recognizable, their own utilization review would carry the heavy end of the pole for the public programs. The model fails to infuse hope for either the quality of beneficiary care or the economy of program operations.

Of course, if Medicare and Medicaid do survive in something resembling the present formulation, instead of the voucher roulette that gleams in the eye of enterprise, there will be, and probably should be, changes in reimbursement practice. One of the things the new force aims at accomplishing, in addition to getting the government off our backs, is getting its hand out of our pockets, and the accepted method for shifting the payment incentive from charge to save is prospective reimbursement. The trials up to now have produced mixed results, but it seems likely nevertheless that the favored maneuver may be a move toward payment by diagnosis-related groups—in the aggregate an organized form of robbing Peter to pay Paul, on the theory that Paul is more efficient than Peter, again in the aggregate, though in the opinion of some whose hospitals have been engaged in the DRG experiments this is not invariably the case. But any system of payment must have its winners and losers, and this one may come as close as any to ensuring that the winners are the brighter, if not always the more deserving.

But it appears that the hospital field is really not that worried about the proposals to scuttle PSRO without anybody knowing who's going to bell the cat for employers and health plans and consumers, or about the likelihood that planning authority will be moved out of the community and into the statehouse, or about the possibility that the laborious business of negotiating approval of Medicare cost reports will be supplanted by the laborious process of negotiating DRG budget reports. The worst uncertainties, the ones that are going to keep hospital people awake all night and their communities confused all day, are not the things that are going out of style but the things that are coming in, and the riddle at the top of the list is, "What happens when medical and hospital services are bought and sold in a free market?" That is to say, of course, a market that is freer than it has been in the past. It is understood all around that "free" in this context is not the "free market" economists talk about. What is intended here is a free market for the anointed—for everybody except the storefront faith healers and psychics and all the other practitioners and assistants we think should be limited or excluded from competing, for the good reason that we consider their qualifications as healers questionable and their services hazardous for our communities, and not for the bad reason that it would cost us some of our revenues to let them compete. But the purity of our motives does not alter the embarrassing circumstance that all our talk about free-market forces means free for us, not them, as Princeton University economist Uwe Reinhardt likes to point out. We want the government off our backs, but not off theirs.

Nevertheless, the idea of competition as an alternative to oppressive regulation is so overwhelmingly attractive to Americans that we are going to find out whether or not the idea works in the market for medical services. In the name of free competition and free-market forces, certainly without reference to and possibly without awareness of the limited or parochial sense of the terms as they are used here, the Congress will enact one or another or some combination of the legislative proposals to stimulate price competition among health insurers, health care providers, and those hybrid insurer-provider constructs that are called simply "health plans" in the proposed legislation, and "health maintenance organizations" by most of the rest of us, and "prepaid group practice" by the few of us who are old enough to remember that they have been around for 50 or 60 years. The big idea is to mandate the offering of several health plans and equalize the tax advantages and employer contributions so that employees could save money by choosing cheaper plans. At the same time, it is expected that health plans would spring up all over the place and shop around for the best prices among hospitals and physician groups, which would then have the incentives to economize that have been missing in the fee-for-service and cost reimbursement health insurance plans that have prevailed up to now. The result of all this competition among providers and health plans for favor among employers and consumers is expected to create a free market for medical services, in contrast to the highly structured and regulated market that has contributed to excesses of facilities, equipment, services, and prices; the free market, its celebrants postulate, will bring down or hold down the costs that all the regulatory efforts of the past decade have so notably failed to do.

It seems a reasonable expectation on the face of it, and there are places where it may work—like Massachusetts, for example, where state rate regulation is so stringent and state payments so stingy that hospitals and doctors are ready to try anything, and Orange County, CA, where the competition among hospitals and doctors and health plans is so frenzied already that nobody would notice the difference. But there are also awesome risks, in California and Massachusetts, and all over. It was in California, as a matter of fact, during the *first* rebirth of enthusiasm for HMOs in the early 1970s, that the state contracted with a number of newly organized health plans to provide services for Medi-Cal beneficiaries, and some of these turned out to be promotional scams, and a lot of people got hurt. So there will have to be regulation of the new health plans; it needn't be oppressive, but it will subtract something more from the freedom of the free market.

Another consideration is the possible damage to the institutions that have made American medicine a world leader—the academic medical centers and teaching hospitals. "Underlying the proposed competitive models is the assumption that hospitals provide a relatively standardized product which is easily identifiable in terms of cost and quality," said John A.D. Cooper, M.D., president of the Association of American Medical Colleges. "This assumption raises several issues for teaching hospitals, which have multiple products benefitting not only the individual patient but society as a whole. Because these activities are expensive, result in higher costs for teaching hospitals, and are presently financed to a large extent through patient care revenues, competitive pricing resulting from the proposed legislation could jeopardize the ability of teaching hospitals to meet their multiple responsibilities in medical education, research technology, tertiary care, and quality care."[1] The Secretary of Health and Human Services has acknowledged the problem and suggested as a possible remedy the creation of a trust fund through which the special needs and expenses of these institutions may be accommodated. This is soothing, but the teaching hospitals are still nervous, and in any event a special trust fund means identifying and qualifying regulations, and another ring around freedom.

The ring around freedom that could be the most difficult of all to deal with, however, is the one doctors and hospitals must impose on themselves if they are to retain the trust of their communities in the era of competition. In the competitive scramble, if price does become a compelling consideration of choice, as the architects of the new order are counting on it to do, the pressures to cut down cost at the expense of quality will be relentless. Under the circumstances, how can communities be confident that their hospitals will come down on the side of safety and quality, instead of economy and price advantage, in the decisions that have to be made every day that nobody on the outside—no consumer, no employer, no health plan entrepreneur—will ever know about?

In the competitive era, the basis for the community's confidence will be what is has always been: trust in the intentions as well as the competence of its doctors and hospitals. Even in a decade characterized by the erosion of public trust in institutions of all kinds, doctors and hospitals have remained relatively unaffected by the growing public cynicism—an often overlooked but significant fact that has been demonstrated repeatedly in public opinion polls and in communities' reactions when their hospitals have been threatened. Maintaining the community's trust isn't just a matter of public or community relations technique, like getting the good stories in the papers and on television and keeping the bad stories out, or like saying "hospital field" instead of "hospital industry." It's a matter of maintaining performance, and maintaining performance under pressure more than anything else is a matter of moral character, of resisting the temptation to shave points off quality to gain points in price when nobody will know the difference.

Nobody will know but the trimmers themselves, and for a time they will have the edge, and then others will think everybody else is doing it so they have to. Trimming is contagious, like lying among competitive salesmen; in time the moral distinction between the hospital mission and the ends of commerce will disappear, and the society will be the loser. It doesn't have to happen that way, of course, and it could happen that way without price competition. But price competition will tend to push in that direction, as a hospital association official unconsciously suggested in a recent publication. "For years our industry idealized the objective 'to provide the highest quality care at the lowest possible cost to the patient,' " he said. "Perhaps at this time our objective may be 'to provide the lowest possible cost to the patient at the highest possible quality level.' " The difference is something to think about.

[1]Panel on Regulation vs. Competition in the Health Care Field, presented at the Blue Cross and Blue Shield Symposium 5, "Health Care in the 80s and Beyond," Chicago: November 20, 1980.

Consumerism:
The Tables Are Turning

March 1981

In the early years of Medicare and Medicaid, before the bloom was off the Great Society and the War on Poverty had ended in stalemate, calls for consumer representation in health affairs were the order of the day. Ralph Nader had shaken up the automobile industry and was busy testifying at congressional hearings and peering down corporate corridors looking for "crime in the suites," and his associates in the Health Research Group were putting together a manual telling consumers what kind of questions to ask their community hospitals. The cities were dotted with Office of Economic Opportunity (OEO) neighborhood clinics, whose consumer representatives or "community advisory committees" had to be in place before the money would start flowing. A Secretary's Task Force on Medicaid and Related Programs recommended broad consumer representation in the formulation and conduct of government health programs and consumer participation in the deliberations of organizations and institutions involved in planning, purchasing, and delivering health services. "One of the basic assumptions underlying this report is that the consumer can be a responsible partner in a system that requires intelligent and caring people to make it work," the task force said, adding that "the consumer can help to identify problems and inadequacies in medical care, can suggest solutions, and can help to design and implement new policy."[1]

It wasn't easy. Roger O. Egeberg, M.D., who was dean of the School of Medicine at the University of Southern California at the time, told a national conference on medical costs how the community advisory committee of the OEO clinic at Watts, in Los Angeles, was organized. "Almost a thousand names were suggested by churches, organizations, Congressmen, supervisors, health departments, and others," he said. "Finally, 18 members were chosen. At the first meeting, they were asked among other things what they thought they needed most in the way of health services for the area. No answers for quite a while. Finally a woman got up and said she thought the most useful thing would be a slab on every corner. A *slab?* 'Yes, a slab to lay people on while they are waiting for the ambulance or the hearse.' Further questioning brought out the fact that this was indeed the concept of medical care of many of these people. One sought it in dire emergency, when death was impending or at least seemed to be around the corner."[2]

Aside from the possibility that the slab proposal may have been a sarcastic appraisal of what was seen as the prevailing professional attitude toward care of the underprivileged, the episode may offer a clue to the difficulties encountered by those who tried to make consumer representation work in health institutions and programs. To begin with, although it was rarely so stated, in the context of the 1960s consumer representation meant representation of the unrepresented, and chiefly representation of and by minorities. This didn't work too badly in the case of the OEO clinics, which were established for the most part to serve poor inner-city populations and usually staffed by young physicians dedicated to serving the poor. In fact, in some OEO clinics in the late 1960s the only way you could tell the doctors from the patients was that the doctors were the ones with the stethoscopes.

Consumer representation in the governance of hospitals was something else. "Health professionals have been reluctant to share decision making in health policy and continue to regard policy making as their traditional domain," the Medicaid Task Force had said, calling a spade a teaspoon. And apart from the disposition of professionals to look upon nonprofessionals as peasants, there was always the problem of selection. What were the criteria for consumer representation on a hospital board of trustees? Obviously, it had to be someone who lived in the community and looked to the hospital for service, but what else? Education had to be considered, but not exclusively, or too many people would be ruled out, and the same thing was true of economic status. A leadership role in some community group was usually considered indicative of desirable qualifications; these people would be familiar with community needs and feelings, and their opinions would be respected. Also, they were visible, and thus easily identifiable as community representatives. So they were the ones most commonly chosen.

Sometimes it worked, but often it didn't, because the qualities that made community leaders effective for other purposes could be inconsistent with hospital goals and methods. The militant tactics that worked well in battles with city officials and landlords and merchants weren't exactly what hospitals had to have for determining consumer needs and shaping services accordingly. The shouting match is rarely an efficient instrument for making policy. Thus while there have been instances of inner-city hospitals whose consumer representative appointments to the board have been successful and resulted in changed procedures and in some cases addition of needed services, for many institutions another kind of representation appeared to accomplish the purpose without risking the disruption that an unfortunate selection might cause.

"There has been a persistent clamor for neighborhood or community or consumer groups to have representation on hospital boards of trustees," Russell A. Nelson, M.D., former president of the Johns Hopkins Hospital, wrote in the report of his study of voluntary teaching hospitals in New York City in 1974. "This occurs because such groups feel excluded from the mechanism of control, without a voice in having their needs met by the institution which is there to serve them. The point is entirely valid. However, it may be that membership on sub-boards and committees that deal directly with management and staff, rather than on the board, is the most effective method by which such groups may be heard. This is particularly important in ambulatory and emergency services, where most of the unsatisfactory conditions exist. If this mechanism is used, trustees should monitor its working routinely to ensure that it is functioning properly."[3]

Nelson also suggested that the deliberations of such a sub-board or committee could be expected to identify consumer representatives who would become suitable trustee candidates and would "bring to trusteeship a dimension that has often been missing: a thoughtful understanding of patient and community needs and feelings and a willingness to listen and learn about the hospital's resources and limitations." The community committee device has proved to be a successful way of accommodating consumer representation in many urban hospitals, and in some cases it has resulted in recruitment of trustees who brought new insights to board discussions of patient care. Among the services that have been introduced as a consequence of such consumer participation, the more common ones have been ombudsmen and patient representatives, alcohol and drug abuse clinics, ambulance service with two-way radio communication, bilingual staffing of emergency and outpatient services, and a variety of patient and public education programs. Some suburban and small-town hospitals have also had community committees, but here the value must be measured largely in terms of public relations rather than substantive contributions to patient care. In the suburban community, particularly, the population is likely to be homogeneous; everybody is a consumer representative, and adding a few more to the board or creating another committee might just add individual opinions without producing anything new.

Of course, the most pervasive form of consumer representation in health affairs in our time has been on health systems agency (HSA) boards, where consumer majorities were mandated by a law that started a lot of arguments, not all settled yet, about who is a consumer and who isn't. Regulators kept insisting that the HSA board should as nearly as possible reflect the composition of the community population—a virtual guarantee of confusion, if not shouting matches. And as might have been expected, requiring a majority of public board members in an activity supported by public funds was also a virtual guarantee that the memberships would be sought by those with axes to grind, and a Gresham's law of public appointments would take over.

Under the circumstances, the remarkable thing is not that so many HSAs have accomplished so little but that some have accomplished something. The argument about whether the whole apparatus should be wiped out or not has already started and is likely to continue for months, with one side claiming it has cost an arm and a leg and hasn't saved a toe, and the other side claiming mythical millions in beds not filled and buildings not built, and neither side able to prove anything. Either way, it will have created a new occupation, the professional health planner, and it will have taught a few thousand consumer board members that there is more to health services than slabs on street corners. These are probably useful results, and in any case the argument will be settled more by political irrelevancies than by informed judgments, and the facts will remain obscure.

Whatever the outcome, the consumer movement didn't begin with the confrontation tactic of Ralph Nader in the 1960s, and it won't die if HSAs should vanish in the 1980s. The consumer confrontation was not unknown in the agoras of ancient Greece, where the pupils of Socrates learned to demand a just price and keep a sharp eye out for adulterated goods and short weights, evils that are still around. Laws aimed at protecting consumers from adulterated foods and drugs were enacted in Great Britain and the United States in the 19th century—a circumstance that may surprise some of today's deregulation enthusiasts who assume that such laws were created *do novo* in our time by a government hell-bent to shackle free enterprise.

These and the similar laws that followed over the years weren't particularly effective, however, and in 1927 U.S. economist Stuart Chase and F.J. Schlink, an engineer associate, wrote a book called *Your Money's Worth,* a study of the National Bureau of Standards, which the authors said was doing a good job of testing goods supplied to government departments. But unfortunately the public had no such protective screen and was getting ripped off, said the book, which became an instant best seller and, as Nader's *Unsafe At Any Speed* did 40 years later, became the forerunner of a generation of reforms and regulations. Among other things, *Your Money's Worth* resulted in Consumers Research, an organization run by Schlink, and, in 1936, Consumers Union, whose stated purpose was "to provide information and counsel relating to consumer goods and services, to give information and assistance on matters relating to expenditures of family income, and to initiate and cooperate with individual and group efforts to create and maintain decent living standards." Consumers Union now has more than two million members and has spawned a number of publications and affiliates, including similar organizations in Britain, France, Germany, Sweden, and Japan.

Growth to two million members in a 40-year period characterized by expansion of population, government, labor, industry, and education might be considered something less than sensational, but the fact is that consumer organizations as such represent only a small fraction of the consumer movement. Labor unions, for example, have accomplished many of the protective and advocacy purposes of consumer organizations over these years. The student movement of the 1960s was in effect a consumer movement, and in many ways the women's movement of the 1970s has had similar goals.

The role of government with respect to the consumer movement and its objectives has been, to state the proposition conservatively, disarranged. The Congress passes laws and establishes regulatory agencies, usually as a response to perceived inequities, to protect citizens as consumers, and over time the agencies take on a life of their own. Usually they are seen by consumers as captives of the industries they were established to regulate, and by the industries as dictatorial and capricious. Both views may be right; in any event, a White House Office of Consumer Affairs (OCA) in recent years has functioned to a large extent as a participant on the consumer's side in regulatory proceedings. "OCA can act on behalf of all consumers to protest proposals by industry and submit evidence that will be considered in the decision-making process," the *Washington Post* said. "Generally, consumers have not been represented in cases before regulatory agencies, although the agencies are supposed to act in the public interest."

Reflecting the antiregulation fever that has been epidemic in Washington and elsewhere for the past year, the Senate last fall was moved to pass an amendment to an appropriations bill prohibiting OCA intervention in regulatory proceedings. Sen. John Danforth (R-MO) called OCA's interventions "an affront to Congress" and said OCA was attempting to assume powers the Congress had rejected when it killed the proposed Consumer Protection Agency bill in 1978.

If the antiregulation fever is bad for consumers, however, it may be good for the consumer movement, for reasons that were explained by William R. Fasse, Ph.D., a member of the steering committee of the Conference of Consumer Organizations, who noted that the number of state and local consumer organizations and public interest groups has been rising steadily. "The basic issue of the consumer movement is the conflict between consumers and sellers in the marketplace," Fasse said. "As long as a marketplace exists, a consumer movement will exist. The movement will take different forms at different times, but it will always be a part of the economy. The activity level of the consumer movement will be in relation to the difference in power between consumers and sellers. An objective analysis of the increases in power of sellers in terms of law, policy, and economic control in the marketplace leads to the conclusion that the consumer movement will be a growth industry in the last two decades of this century."[4]

The essence of the consumer movement in our time has been populism, an attempt to redress the imbalance of economic power between seller and buyer—that is, between business and industry as sellers and the rank and file of the people as buyers—and the strategy of the movement has been to arm the people with information and enlist the power of government on the people's side. The anomaly of the consumer movement in health care today is that the roles are being reversed: Increasingly, business and industry and government are buyers of health services on behalf of the people, and the increases in the power of buyers in terms of law, policy, and economic control in the health care marketplace lead to the conclusion that the consumer movement as we have known it in the past may have a diminished function in the coming decade. The greater need may be for a provider movement.

[1]Department of Health, Education, and Welfare, Report of the Task Force on Medicaid and Related Programs, Washington, DC: U.S. Government Printing Office, June, 1970.

[2]Egeberg, R., Organization for the Delivery of Care, in U.S. Dept. of Health, Education, and Welfare, Report of the National Conference on Medical Costs, June 27-28, 1967, Washington, DC: U.S. Government Printing Office, 1968.

[3]Nelson, R. The Governance of Voluntary Teaching Hospitals in New York City, New York: Josiah Macy Jr. Foundation, 1974.

[4]Fasse, W., COCO Intercom. October 1980.

Comfort and Consequences

June 1976

Alex Comfort, the British biologist, was an authority on aging before he became an authority on sex and will probably remain an authority on aging after he has become a former authority on sex, because biological research is the whole base for his authority on aging, whereas the research base of his authority on sex has a superstructure of popular fancy that could be toppled at any time by a new writer with a new angle, or position. For the last year, at any rate, Dr. Comfort has been a Senior Fellow at the Center for the Study of Democratic Institutions in Santa Barbara, Calif., where he was recently interviewed by another Senior Fellow, Harvey Wheeler, a writer and political science professor who appeared to know what Dr. Comfort was talking about as they discussed the aging process and chatted about such things as DNA, RNA, cell reproduction, immunocytes, mutagens, cross-linking agents, antioxidants, enzyme-inducers, and DDT, a familiar substance that Dr. Comfort said may turn out to have some life-prolonging properties.

However it may be brought about, Dr. Comfort remains confident that the aging process can be retarded, not only so as to prolong life but also to make people younger longer. "If we were to prolong life by the expedient we're talking about, slowing down aging," he explained, "the effect wouldn't be visible in looking at the community, because a person of 70 might look as if he were 50 and would have the same health as if he were 50." While this might not be an unmixed blessing for the rest of the population, and perhaps especially not for 50-year olds, it would surely be welcomed by the aged themselves, who have been identified increasingly in recent years as an oppressed minority. "The elderly have become a social and political problem," Mr. Wheeler said. "To put it another way," he added, "they've become a social and political force. We see all kinds of evidence of it. We have a new word—'agism'—a counterpart of sexism. We think of it primarily with regard to discrimination against the elderly."[1]

If the aged have indeed become a social and political force without any help from antioxidants and DDT, they may readily run the rest of us out of house room when these and other retardants, or putative retardants, get going. The United States ia already included in the list of what demographers call "mature populations," along with such venerable company as Finland and Poland, and in fact, according to the 1971 edition of the "United Nations Demographic Yearbook" we are on the threshold of joining Italy, Switzerland, France, Germany and Sweden, among others, in the group labeled "aged populations." In the demographic culture a nation is seen as young if its population age 65 and over is less than 4 per cent of the total, youthful at 4 to 7 per cent, mature at 7 to 10, and aged from 10 to wherever, so the chances are that we have already left maturity behind and joined the early elderly, as it has been called. For a population, the process of aging begins with declining mortality in the early years of life, followed by declining fertility rates and declining death rates. "In societies with aged populations the older generation differs from the younger in many ways other than simply age," said Donald O. Cowgill, Ph.D., a professor of sociology at the University of Missouri and a certified authority on the demography of aging. "The older generation has a higher ratio of females and of widows. The elderly have less formal education; they have lower incomes, and they are less mobile. Older populations also differ from the younger ones in marital status. Given the sex ratios and differential mortality rates, one should expect more widows than widowers in the older population."[2] In the U.S., for example, 52 per cent of the females age 65 and over were widows in 1970, but only 17 per cent of the males of the same age were widowers, and unless Dr. Comfort should find a magic that works better for males that females, it would appear that the old women will outnumber the old men by increasing margins as the years go on—a circumstance that would have obvious significance for institutional facilities and services.

But it isn't necessarily so, according to Dr. Cowgill. "There is nothing inevitable about the process," he said. "There are many developments which would prevent or reverse it, but most of these are in the nature of disasters—such as nuclear warfare, widespread famine, widespread lethal pollution, or a new virulent epidemic disease—which would reverse the worldwide downward trend in mortality rates. However, if we avoid such disasters and fertility rates are reduced, this will amount to completion of the transition, and it will inevitably result in the aging of the population." What happens then is uncertain, it is acknowledged. "The social consequences of demographic aging are exceedingly complex," Dr. Cowgill said. "Since such demographic aging is an entirely new phenomenon—most of it having occurred during the last century—it should not be surprising that traditional cultures provided no ready-made modes of adjustment to the presence of such a high proportion of older people in the population. Nor should it surprise us that there have been some strains and problems in the adjustment."

As everybody knows, the strains result from the fact that we encourage old people not to work by offering them retirement benefits, and then reject them as an unproductive burden on the society—a process that must have seemed logical at the time it was named 'social security" but appears less so today. "I'm against any compulsory retirement if it means throwing somebody out of a useful life in the community," said Dr. Comfort. "I think that one point in favor of the longer life span, if we get it, is that it would complete the two-style pattern of living which we're beginning to get. There is a whole mass of socially useful activities, and I don't mean just knitting socks or seeing kids across the road, that old people can and should be doing. We have a lovely example in wartime Britain when all the old unemployables came back and did all their own jobs again for years with complete success because the younger men were in the services."

The example suggests a solution for our time: Keep the old people at their own jobs and let the young people, who don't think much of working anyway, have that whole mass of socially useful activities. If they want to, let them knit socks and see kids across the roads. The only trouble is that with everybody running around looking 50 we aren't going to be able to tell which is which. As Mr. Wheeler said, "By and large, people behave the way we tell them we expect them to. We used to tell elderly people that we expected them to act old, and so they went around acting old. Now we tell them they're supposed to act like

Cary Grant and J. Strom Thurmond and Justice Douglas. Sure enough, that's the way they're trying to behave."

Maybe the only sensible thing to do is send Dr. Comfort to New Guinea, where the percentage of the population over age 65 is 1.1.

[1]Center Report, Center for the Study of Democratic Institutions, June, 1974.

[2]Cowgill, Donald O., Ph.D., The Aging of Populations and Societies, The Annals of the American Academy of Political and Social Science, September, 1974.

The Bed You Shrink May Be Your Own

May 1978

Tucked away among the standard articles in the Sunday newspaper supplement about an instant millionaire, a TV comedienne, and a native village in the Amazon jungle was an interview with a retired business executive who expanded on the joys of Life in the Golden Years. What did he consider to be the elements of successful aging? the reporter wanted to know. Good health, certainly, a loving family, useful and interesting work of some kind, and lively companions were the prescription. The executive's wife was present at the interview, and the reporter asked if she had anything to add. "Yes," she said. "Bring money."

It's a point that is often overlooked by those who write and lecture about old age, and, in fact, it was rather glossed over in that most celebrated of all treatises on the subject, Cicero's *De Senectute*. "In abject poverty old age cannot be easy to bear even for a true philosopher," acknowledged Cicero, who died when he was 63 and must therefore have had only limited first-hand knowledge of aging. Nevertheless, he considered that there were compensations for such obvious complaints as diminished vigor, fewer pleasures, and approaching death, and as evidence he cited the career of Cato the Elder, who had remained a formidable power in Rome until his death at 85. Like most essays on aging, *De Senectute* offers more comfort for the young than for the old. "Cicero tried to make poor, disappointed, frail people satisfied with old age because Cato, rich, elevated in position, strong and well, found it tolerable," one critic said, and other writers have been falling into the same trap ever since.

A notable exception in our time is Hugh Downs, the TV reporter and entertainer who has been devoting a measurable share of his time to studying the problems of aging and helping the aged. "The importance of material security is somehow always underestimated by younger people," he said recently. "This shows up in the surprise we feel that older people attach such importance to their financial condition. In a physical parallel, you will become much more fearful of falling down if you have doubts about your ability to get back up. Money becomes more important when you can't go out easily and earn more, particularly if you feel you could but society discourages or prohibits it. We have the old who get poor and the poor who get old. It doesn't matter in the end by which route you arrive at being old and poor, money can become very important."

Second only to lack of money among the hardships the aged encounter in a world that is indifferent, if not hostile, is lack of occupation. In her monumental book, *The Coming of Age,* the French writer Simone de Beauvoir reported a survey revealing that, in addition to doing household chores, old people spent a large share of their time sitting in the sun in good weather and looking out the window on cold or rainy days. In America, watching television is a favored pastime in all kinds of weather, but anybody who has spent more than a few minutes viewing daytime TV must know that it is more ataractic than engaging. "Idleness can cause loss of identity, and this in turn can give rise to depression and psychosomatic ills," John H. Budd, M.D., a past president of the American Medical Association, said at a 1974 AMA conference on problems of the aged, where he also referred to an AMA study that found compulsory retirement and artificial barriers to employment based on age to be primary factors in the deterioration of health. "Among the old, loneliness is a frequent companion of idleness," Dr. Budd said. "We can see it every day on faces in the street, the store, the park, yet we underestimate its prevalence and its effects. Most of us assume that the old can always find some kind of association—an institutional home or a retirement community, if not a circle of friends and relatives. The truth is that a fourth of the aged population lives alone or with nonrelatives. Only one in 20 lives in an institution. Many of the ills affecting older people are the product of emotional complications that disturb normal physiological processes, intensify disease processes, and interfere with healing. Encouraging older persons to assume functioning, valuable roles in the family and community will reduce their emotional problems and improve their general health."

Given these basic insecurities, it was not especially comforting for the aged to learn that the federal government is already spending nearly one-third of its budget on services for the elderly and their dependents, and the proportion is expected to continue rising. "There has been a tremendous graying of the federal budget over the past 10 years," Joseph Califano said when he was HEW secretary, exercising his gift for language calculated to set off a nervous train of thought among those likely to be affected by whatever it is he may be saying. HEW spends $90 billion a year in Social Security payments, mostly for the elderly, $35 billion for Medicare and Medicaid services, and $2 billion more for welfare and special programs, Califano reported. Other federal services pay another $26 billion in civil service, military, and railroad pensions, and by 1989 as much as 45 percent of the total budget may be spent for all these services if the trend continues, Califano estimated. For example, he said, half of all the money for Medicaid goes for long-term care, and thus the growing population of aged persons takes an increasing share of the Medicaid total. Economists have figured out that today there are three members of the working force to pay the taxes needed to support one retiree, but if the shifting composition of the population continues the way it has been going for the past generation, the time could come when the formula will be one worker, one gaffer. In fact, General Motors has estimated that its four-to-one ratio of workers to retirees on pension will be approaching two-to-one by the early 1990s. "We're building one hell of a burden for our future workers," GM's Victor Zink has commented, and a California economist suggested that what is bad for General Motors may be bad for the country: "There is a danger that in the future workers will just say, 'We've had it. We will no longer support all these old people.' "

What old people? U.S. Department of Commerce population projections indicate that the percentage of the population over age 65, which was 10.5 last year, will increase to 11.7 in 1990, to 14.6 in 2020, and to 17.0 in 2030, by which time it could go as high as 20.9 percent, depending on what happens to the fertility rate in the meantime. And whatever the population over age 65 may become, the segments over ages 75 and 85 will have increased at substantially faster rates. That means we may have 50 million over age 65 in another 50 years. Twenty-one million of these would be over 75, and four or five million over 85. The morbidity rates in these age groups for cardiovascular diseases, influenza and pneumonia, neoplasms, diabetes, renal disease, and fractures, among other causes, suggest that it will take all the hospital beds we have now to take care of the aged alone, and twice the present number of nursing home beds to provide for those with chronic illnesses. It's a thought we should keep in mind as we go about the business of shrinking the health care system.

Of course, it might not work out exactly that way. It might be worse. In a recent book, Albert Rosenfeld, science editor of *Saturday Review* and adjunct professor of human biological chemistry and genetics at the University of Texas Medical Branch at Galveston, reported some of the studies now going on in gerontological research centers around the world. Scientists are not given generally to wild speculation about the probable results of their work, so Rosenfeld considered it remarkable that many of them felt free to tell him of their confidence that it is just a question of time until they learn enough about the aging process to ensure that it can be retarded significantly—some said by the end of the century, others perhaps a generation beyond that. Rosenfeld himself saw several lines of investigation converging in what he called a "unified field theory" of aging. "... genetic switching, cross-linkage, free radicals, auto-immunity, somatic mutations. I will venture to predict that by the year 2025, if research proceeds at reasonable speed, most of the major mysteries of the aging process will have been solved and the solutions adopted as part of conventional biomedical knowledge; and that some of the solutions will by then already have come into practical use to stave off the ravages of senescence."[1]

Considering that all the beds are going to be filled anyway, the queues at the hospital door might not be that much longer. If the aging process can indeed be slowed down, your 75-year-olds of the 21st century are going to be as healthy and energetic as our 50-year-olds are today. They will be jogging in the parks, and those old folks we'll be expanding our hospitals to accommodate will be in their early 100s and complaining about the high cost of nursing home care for their parents. In any case, it may readily be beds for the well that worry us most. Space, food, energy, and jobs may all be in limited supply. "Certainly the first resource we are running out of is food," said Sicco Mansholt, Dutch agricultural economist who was president of the

European Common Market. "The second disaster will be the destruction of an ecological balance. The third is linked up with the environment, and will represent the running out of energy. Over the next 15 or 20 years this planet has to meet its greatest difficulties, but it seems quite unprepared to squarely face them."[2]

Many economists, industrialists, and politicians in the industrial nations consider that Mansholt and those who share his views are doomsday alarmists. Economic growth will make available the resources to guard against its own ill effects, in this cheerier outlook. Still others consider that the problem will not be the shortage of resources but management of the shortage. "If in fact the limits of growth become apparent, then I believe there will be a very significant social upheaval in the industrial societies, as the great mass of people who are underprivileged, oppressed in many ways, recognize that they no longer have any reason to accept a system which is prejudiced against them," said Noam Chomsky, the Massachusetts Institute of Technology professor of linguistics who has opinions on everything from syntax to sin and is probably without peer as a gadfly's gadfly. "I cannot predict the outcome of that kind of struggle," he added.[3]

Nobody can. But whether our children's children's children live in a world of peace and plenty made possible by technologies we haven't yet dreamed of, or whether they must survive clinging to whatever may be left them from the upheaval foreseen by Chomsky, the changed composition of the population will make their society very different from ours—possibly restoring some of the respect for age that was evident in ancient Eastern cultures and still had traces in early America but has vanished in our time as we elbow the elderly out of their jobs, and often their homes, to make room for the young. This practice will not be practical, or even possible, when there are 50 million of them. The political influence of the aged, inchoate and barely felt today, can be expected to become a powerful and directed force in future generations. The movement to raise the compulsory retirement age from 65 to 70 has been fueled by the desire to save Social Security funds, not to let old people keep on working, but a militant multitude of 50 million might take a notion to turn the Social Security system upside down and support the young so the old can keep their jobs, and their power, and their money. Whatever they do about jobs, however, they're going to need, and get, a larger share of the health care resources. If there is a single industry around that is a dead sure thing for growth for the next 50 years, that is it.

[1]Rosenfeld, A., Prolongevity: A Report on the Scientific Discoveries Now Being Made About Aging and Dying, and Their Promise of an Extended Life Span—Without Old Age, New York: Alfred A. Knopf, 1976.

[2]Oltmans, W.L., ed., On Growth: The Crisis of Exploding Population and Resource Depletion, New York: G.P. Putnam's Sons, 1974.

[3]ibid.

What Old People Want:
More Work, Less Talk

May 1980

A headline in a recent issue of *Forbes* magazine might readily be considered the core concept of a new mode of conservative thought about old people. "The myth is that they're sunk in poverty," this said. "The reality is that they're living well. The trouble is there are too many of them."[1]

The article, one of several that have appeared in magazines and newspapers in the past few months, dismissed the notion that old people on fixed incomes are having a hard time made harder by inflation. "In fact, that image of poverty is false," the *Forbes* writer said. "On the whole, America's retired aren't doing badly at all, better in fact than many of their working sons and daughters." As evidence, he cited the case of a Florida couple that plays tennis every day when they aren't busy taking bridge and dancing lessons; an old lady in Massachusetts who lives in subsidized housing on Social Security and a modest retirement income and saves $100 a month because there's nothing for her to buy but food, and a 73-year-old in Pasadena who avoids common shares at 7 percent and buys Treasury bills that pay 11. The clincher for *Forbes,* whose argument is that we're already spending too much on the aged and we'd better hold back because there are going to be a lot more of them in a few years, is the case of a West Virginia coal miner who retired at 55 after two heart attacks and is getting $471 a month in Social Security disability. $329 from his United Mine Workers pension, and $381 from the government in benefits for black-lung disease. "That adds up to $14,172 a year, largely tax free, and more than the straight time take-home wages that he earned when working," said *Forbes,* obviously distressed about such extravagance. "He owns his house free and clear, as many

151

elderly do, and the car is paid for, too. He also owns a paid-for 29-foot pontoon boat tied up on the Kanawha River only a stone's throw from his backyard."

Not to worry, *Forbes*. With two heart attacks and black lung, he isn't going to be living it up long enough to use that much of your tax money. And when that old lady in Massachusetts has to go to a nursing home, Medicaid will make her go through her bank account before they start leaning on you to help pay for her care.

Without being quite so barefaced about it, a lot of people are worried about the rising cost of Social Security, Medicare, and other benefits for the aged, and are looking with concern at the population projections that show how much the burden is going to increase over coming generations. Under the circumstances, the effort to picture 80-year-olds engaging in riotous living at public expense was probably inevitable and may be put down not so much to insensitivity or cruelty as to a planned public relations maneuver aimed at building political pressure opposing any added benefits. Happily for the aged, not all of whom possess paid-for 29-foot pontoon boats, they have enough votes already to make it politically imprudent to propose snatching benefits away, as one of this year's candidates discovered last time around, and enough votes up to now to stall serious consideration of an amendment that would require old people to pay income taxes on their Social Security.

But the O.P. vote (the term is used in a *Saturday Review* article and reported as common in Florida, where old people and young people are said to be practically at war over government benefits) hasn't been strong enough to make it possible for the old to keep on working without sacrificing Social Security, as they can do under the programs for the aged in most European countries. In *The Coming of Age,* the seminal book on how society treats old people, Simone de Beauvoir reported that as many as two-thirds of eligible pensioners in some countries keep on working and paying taxes, a policy that relieves some of the burden on government and elevates pensioners above the dependency level. The reason it isn't done here is thought to be that business executives are worried that they'll lose talented young people who will see their careers blocked, and worried about the problems that will come up if older workers can't handle their jobs, and worried because unknown retirement dates would mess up manpower planning.

The lid on these and other horrors associated with keeping old people on the premises was lifted a little last year when the age for compulsory retirement was raised from 65 to 70 years. It will be some time before there can be any assessment of what happens, but there are signs suggesting that the business world may survive. Thus a Chicago manufacturing firm that never did have mandatory retirement and has two top executives over 70, phenomena that may not be completely unrelated, had reported earlier that "the company grew up with the philosophy that a person should be able to be a productive employee for as long as he or she wants to work. It's ability that counts, and you don't suddenly lose it when you turn 65."[2] The company has made its policy work for 40 years without coming apart, it is reported, and it seems likely that there may be sensible solutions to the problems that are making so many executives nervous. "Many young people are looking for a pre-planned career today, but we won't promise that," the firm's personnel manager said. "Instead, we show people that we recognize ability and promote from within." So what happens when the path to promotion is clogged up by an old-timer who is doing his job and won't go quietly? "Young people react differently. Some resent it, but others think it's great that a company wouldn't try to force someone out just because of age," an industrial psychologist said. "I'm working with one client that's considering opening a machine shop manned exclusively by people over 65. There's a shortage of skilled machinists, and we're hoping to attract people back to work. They may not want to work 40 hours a week, or 50 weeks a year. With the shortage of skilled people, it could help fill critical manpower needs."

It could also help fill a lot of old people's cupboards. What most of them need most is not dancing lessons, but income. Social Security is "indexed to inflation," but the index is losing the footrace, and while many corporations have made an effort to increase pensions, the increases have been infrequent and small, while inflation is constant and terrifying. Those who think the aged live it up and laugh at the working stiffs carrying the heavy end of the pole like to point out that the number of elderly poor has been decreasing for the past 20 years and is now only 14 percent of the over-65 population. But the definition of poor—under $4,000 a year for two—doesn't comprehend the reality that you can go hungry on twice that today. Food stamps and Medicare, also targets for the look-how-good-they-have-it crowd, are a great help for millions, but these are also shrinking currencies. "Medical costs . . . for the elderly are covered to a great extent by the government's Medicare program, by private insurance or, for the poorest, by Medicaid, another government program," *Forbes* says. "There are extra privileges available to the elderly: tax breaks, cheaper bus fares, local rent subsidies, commissary privileges for the retired military which mean cut-rate prices." Nobody over 65 is going to downgrade Medicare, even while wrestling with its inscrutable forms, but the fact is that it pays just 41 percent of total beneficiary health care costs now, as premiums, deductibles, and coinsurance payments have gone up, and provides only sharply limited benefits in nursing homes, where the needs are often greatest. Medicaid picks up the nursing home burden for many—but only *after* they have exhausted their savings and spent down to the point where they can't afford not to be in a nursing home. Some logic.

The thing that makes *Forbes* wake up at night and cry, and then go down to the office in the morning and write articles about old people and their pontoon boats, is not just what today's benefits are costing the taxpayers, or even what it would cost to fulfill the promises of Medicare and Medicaid and keep Social Security within shouting distance of inflation. The thing that induces panic is what it is going to cost to do any of these things in another generation or so when there will be 55 millions over age 65 and half that many over 75 and the Social Security tax, with present benefits, would be 25 percent of the payroll, and the political muscle of old people may have got to the point where it could threaten the political muscle of industry and money. "Do we throw up our hand in despair? Do we turn to euthanasia for the over-70?" *Forbes* asks. "The situation isn't that bad," it adds hastily, putting down panic. "If there are no easy answers, there are some paths we can follow."

One recommended path would be to encourage people to save for their own retirement, which *Forbes* thinks could be done if it weren't for government tax policy and inflation resulting in "declining savings, declining investment, declining productivity"—a line of thought something like one of Premier Khrushchev's old Russian sayings: "If my grandmother had wheels, she would be a troika." Another measure would be to "curb actual and potential abuses." *Forbes* is convinced there are "massive abuses in so-called disability pensions"—a cheap shot in the absence of any evidence suggesting what the nature of the so-called abuses might be. The most sensible proposal, here and elsewhere, is to encourage old people to keep on working and find ways to make it easy for them, and for their employers. For many, that might be lighter work loads and shorter schedules, or it might be relief—on a sliding scale according to age after 65, say—on income and Social Security taxes, for both employer and employee.

The supposition all along has been that most men and women can't wait until retirement so they can quit working, sleep late, and go fishing, or gardening, or riding around in their trailers, or pontoon boats, or whatever. Of course, millions of them have done just that, many taking advantage of whatever early retirement options their employers may have offered, selling their homes, and moving to Florida or Arizona. But after a few weeks of fishing, or gardening, or shuffle board, they begin to wonder if this was what they really wanted to do. A Duke University Longitudinal Study of Aging has found that "it's not how many friends you have or how you interact with your family that contributes to successful aging, but whether you maintain your activity outside this immediate circle," Dr. Erdman Palmore, professor of medical sociology who directed the study, reported. "People who remain physically active and continue to participate in outside organizations are far more likely to age successfully than those who don't. It may be that just sitting around contributes to depression either directly or indirectly." It can be argued that there has to be a middle ground between working and just sitting around, but the evidence suggests that full-time hobbies and amusements cloy; for many old people in those sun-belt senior citizens' ghettos, the high point of the week is when they call home to find out how things are going back at the plant they couldn't wait to get away from.

But that isn't the main point. The main point is that they need the money, and for those who are willing, the best way to get it may be work. The problem is going to be, if it isn't already, jobs. Manpower theorists are worried because there isn't enough work to go around now, and there is a growing body of opinion among economists and a surprisingly large segment of the public, hotly denied by business and political pietists, that it is no longer sensible to assume continuation of the economic growth that has kept unemployment at manageable limits in the past. "The public is aware of what it regards as a change for the worse in the country's economic circumstances," says the report of a monumental study of current American attitudes, beliefs, and values.[2] "From an expectation of steady growth, ever increasing abundance, continuing improvement in the individual's standard of living, stable prices, and jobs for all who want to work, the majority has shifted ground to expect instead economic instability, recession, depression, continued inflation, joblessness, and shortages."[3] The changing outlook is especially shocking to the old, who are not notably comforted to be referred to as "senior citizens"—an evasive locution whose use suggests that "old" and "aged" are terms of opprobrium. "Suppose someone has lived for years with the expectation that his retirement will be economically secure, and then learns with pained surprise that it will not be," Yankelovich and Lefkowitz say in their report. "If an economically secure retirement is as important to him as it is to most Americans, it will typically take a long time and much anguish to work through the shock of the new circumstance and adapt to it realistically."

The social research data indicate that the aged are not alone in their disillusionment and fear, the investigators report: "When Americans are asked in national polls to describe those elements they believe are most disruptive to a stable life, they include a scarcity of essential resources, mounting personal debt, unjustified corporate profits, the high cost of medical treatment, hazardous working conditions, deterioration of the environment, excessive and wasteful government spending, and the dangers posed by certain forms of technology, particularly nuclear energy. But the one concern that always tops the list is inflation . . . Inflation is now a given in our society; we don't ask whether there will be inflation, we ask how much. After a decade of rising inflation rates, most Americans don't believe they can win the battle against inflation."

Believing they can't win, a large number of Americans—according to Yankelovich a majority, have quit trying and are willing to settle for something less: the growing conviction that what is regarded as a nose-to-the-grindstone way of life with its hard work, its unquestioning loyalty to employers, and its suppression of desires that conflict with obligations to others is too high a price to pay for material success; the feeling that we have devoted too much of our time and attention in this country to the task of how to make a living and not enough to the question of how to live; the belief that what counts most in life is to keep growing as an individual. "Most people appear unsure of these new beliefs and are torn between the old philosophy and the new one," the survey report concludes. "The new values are now merging with the fear of economic instability. A new synthesis is forming that meshes three elements: the pursuit of economic stability, even at the cost of reduced consumption, with more modest material expectations and with the drive to establish maximum control over one's own life and destiny. The combination of these elements creates a novel American outlook."

Like most new ideas and attitudes, this novel American outlook, if it is to be believed, has to be more characteristic of the young than it is of the old, and in the years ahead it may prove to be the young who are willing to sit around on their assets and unemployment insurance while the old work and pay taxes. Employers who are tired of young workers who watch clocks, shun responsibility, and lie about days off may be persuaded in time that there is something to be said for keeping or hiring men and women in their 60s and 70s who are glad to have jobs and are past caring about promotions and privileges, and won't consider that mean or messy tasks are beneath their dignity. With more than their share of mean and messy tasks, hospitals could take the lead in a movement to give old people jobs. In addition to believing in the vanishing idea that work is a virtue *per se,* we may be the last to cling to the old-fashioned notion that there is something distinctive and noble, and worth cherishing, about the hospital's place in society.

[1]Flint, J., The Old Folks, Forbes, February 18, 1980.

[2]Nekvasil, C.A., Then What? TWA Ambassador, March, 1978.

[3]Yankelovich, D., and Lefkowitz, B., The Public Debate on Growth: Preparing for Resolution. Prepared as a Mitchell Prize Award paper for the Third Biennial Woodlands Conference on Growth Policy, Houston: October 1979.

Hospitals Could
Provide the
Voluntary Initiative

December 1980

The certainty that the pressure on hospital costs will continue unabated was in evidence throughout the long, lukewarm election year: Whenever the reporters and heavy thinkers of press and television took a breather from telling us, syllable by syllable, what the candidates said as they kept shooting each other's kneecaps, we got another horror story about a hospital bill or a doctor's fee, plus a cartoon repeating one or another of the tired old jokes of the same genre, plus an editorial going over the well-worn statistics, expressing shock, and calling for remedial action. In one of only a few departures from the familiar script, a noted columnist pointed out that the cost of health care this year was expected to reach 9.7 percent of gross national product, or nearly twice the amount of the defense budget. He forgot to say why that was bad.

Whether it is or not, there can't be much doubt that the efforts to contain costs, voluntary and involuntary, will keep the heat on hospital trustees, managers, and physicians. Rates of payment by third parties will be held down, and standards of medical necessity will be tightened up. Beds and populations will be counted and recounted; politicians and bureaucrats will play the planning guidelines like the national anthem. As soon as the Congress gets organized, those competition bills will get combed out and brushed up, and some kind of competition construct will become law and beget regulations.

Given the circumstance and the likelihood that all these forces will keep rising, enlivened by intramural competition, it may be considered astonishing that so many hospital trustees and executives have been enlarging the focus of hospital responsibility to comprehend the well in addition to the sick populations of their communities, and initiating programs of preventive services, health promotion, health education, and physical fitness. Actually, however, the old pressures and the new horizons are not totally unrelated phenomena. For several years now it has been accepted wisdom that the cost crunch will never be relieved unless more is done to keep the population healthy, and while there are some questions about the sanity of those who consider that keeping people well is a proper function of institutions that don't get paid unless people are sick, there are many who believe that the goal of everything hospitals and doctors do is healthy people, and if it makes as much sense to keep them healthy as it does to get them there, why shouldn't hospitals and doctors get paid for doing both—especially when nobody else knows how? And it may be that the greater number of hospital boards and executives who are cranking up health promotion activities have simply figured that with the cost lid coming down on acute care they had better find some new things to do and get paid for, and this is it. Some of them call it marketing hospital services, which sounds more like cigar stores, and some call it offering new services to the community, which sounds more like hospitals. Whatever they call it, trustees looking for opportunities to add new services have seen health promotion as a logical extension of resources already at hand, and programs have been springing up all over the country, initiated by hospitals of all sizes and types, in all kinds of communities.

Getting paid for these programs is something else. Third parties, whose subscription rates or premiums are based on estimates of the number of people who get sick or hurt, are not notably enthusiastic about trying to finance services for the well population, and while government is pushing health promotion with the right hand in the Surgeon General's office, the left hand in HCFA is slamming the door on the idea that Medicare and Medicaid ought to pay for this kind of nonsense. So for the time being, at least, hospitals going in for expensive health promotion programs have to look for support from industry, which has been willing to pay for almost anything that offers some promise of improving productivity and cutting down the awesome expense of employees' health insurance, and from foundation grants, donors, and individual participants in the programs, who may be the most reliable source for the long term: People who care enough about their health to quit smoking or do pushups ought to be willing to pay somebody to teach them how and keep them at it. Lacking any of these resources, hospitals can always get something back by the method that has paid a lot of medical and nursing education and health education expenses in the past—what some hospital treasurers call "creative cost accounting."

Meanwhile, there are some other service opportunities that individuals and families might readily be willing to pay for themselves—and already do where they can find satisfactory providers, which isn't easy to do. Especially in cities, some hospitals have organized home health care teams to provide needed services for old people who aren't sick enough for Medicare or poor enough for Medicaid but don't need to be in nursing homes and couldn't afford it if they did. Except in suburban communities where young families are the rule, there aren't many places lacking old people who need some kind of home service. More often than not, medical or nursing care is not required: It doesn't take an advanced degree to run errands or make beds or cook meals, or simply to look in and make certain there is no need for a doctor or nurse. One of the nation's leading authorities on aging, Robert Binstock, Ph.D., of Brandeis University, has estimated that families are providing 80 percent of all the social and support services needed by the aged. In many cases families see to these needs because there is nobody else around to do it, he suggested, and families would be glad to have a reliable resource to turn to—and pay. Another noted authority at Brandeis, James J. Callahan Jr., Ph.D., sees these support services as a possibility for development by prepayment and health insurance organizations, and some of them are investigating the feasibility of offering such services as insurance benefits. There may also be an opportunity here for hospitals. For many it would be simply an extension of existing home care or social service operations, but in every case the hospital has the organization, management, and local or community orientation required to estimate the need and test the response.

Ellen Winston, Ph.D., a sociologist who is secretary of the National Council on Aging, has classified the services needed by older adults as including information and referral services, protective services, services to enable persons to remain in or return to their homes or communities, services to meet health needs, homemaker services, legal services, and services to improve living arrangements and enhance activities of daily living, including improved opportunities for social and community participation. "In addition," she has concluded, "many special services have been developed for older adults directly tailored to needs associated with the frailties and disabilities of advanced age."[1]

Winston also emphasized the essentiality of having the services provided by people who are interested in their quality and acceptability. "No service at all is preferable to services poorly rendered," she said. "In working with frail and disabled older adults, one is involved with a highly vulnerable group. Special precautions to guarantee a high quality of service are important, yet there has been a glaring lack of concern for qualitative measures. It is alway surprising to find services of many types developed on an *a priori* basis, instead of turning to tested experience and carefully adhering to such standards as do exist."

Sometimes these services are not just *a priori* but profiteery. In Chicago, Los Angeles, and elsewhere, investigators have discovered so-called not-for-profit agencies that turned out to be screens for money-making scams, billing Medicaid for home care and homemaker services that were deficient or fictitious. In some cases, the same groups were found to be operating under several different names. While there are profit-making corporations that provide competent and conscientious home care and homemaker services, there are also some that are less than satisfactory, and hospital ownership or sponsorship could assure older adults and their families of reliability as well as competence. "Matching the service to the individual in terms of what, how, and by whom rendered can be crucial in determining if a given service is acceptable," Winston said.

It isn't likely that hospitals everywhere are going to jump at the chance to organize homemaking and hand-holding services for the aged, but those that do seem certain to find it a source of revenue that will grow with the increasing numbers of old people in the population, and a priceless means of renewing the hospital's image as an indispensable community service institution—a position that has been threatened, if not lost, in a time characterized by government entitlements, financial pressures, and public criticism. It might also be the precursor of another role that hospitals have generally shunned in the past but that could be the solution to today's problems of excess capacity and the beginning of a new era of expansion: the hospital as a center of health and social services for the aged. One of the few things about the economy that can be predicted with certainty for the coming decades is that old people will be the ascendant group in the population. Ageism will disappear from the society with the growing realization that everybody ages, and, as the biologist Alex Comfort has said, "discriminating against old people is like slashing our own tires."

The opportunity for hospitals is obtrusively evident. The basic needs for the ailing aged are for nursing home and home nursing services. Already old people are stacked up in hospitals for want of acceptable nursing home accommodations, and stacked up in nursing homes for want of acceptable home nursing service. The basic needs for people over age 75 who are neither sick nor rich nor blessed with families that are nearby and attentive are for homemaking and home-visiting services. Hospitals could provide all these services, and something more that is going to become a desperate need in the years ahead. Gerontological research centers are focusing on studies of senile dementia, the chief cause of long-term or permanent institutionalization, when families can no longer provide the care that is needed and it is unsafe to leave patients unattended. It is now possible to distinguish between dementias caused by organic brain disease that is irreversible and those presenting similar behavior and loss of function resulting from causes that are treatable, so patients can be rehabilitated and trained to get along, and get around, with minimum supervision, if not complete independence. In nursing centers at or closely allied to hospitals this kind of rehabilitation care and training could be provided, and a sizeable fraction of the one and a half million patients now in nursing homes could be returned to their homes, or to residential facilities where the needed supervision could be provided at a fraction of the cost of nursing home care. Without the voluntary initiative that hospitals could provide, none of this will happen. Patients will be stacked up in institutions in increasing numbers, and the taxpayers will have to choose between accepting the burden and slashing their own tires.

PATIENTS
AND PUBLICS

The Unchanging Dimensions

May 1972

A reporter who has spent the greater part of a working life-time peering at, or into, hospitals and hospital affairs had occasion not long ago, for only the second time in 30 years, to carry on his observations from that instructive and illuminating, if not always informed and impartial, vantage point, the hospital bed. In the current instance, as in a similar occurrence 12 years ago, the opportunity came about as the result of an accident that required hospitalization beginning at the emergency room. In both cases the injuries were essentially the same: fracture of the tibia, multiple in the first episode 12 years ago and only a single crack this time around, but in the same battered bone—a circumstance that contributed overtones of *deja vu* to the second experience.

In comparing hospital phenomena seen and felt during the two hospital stays, the observer had to keep in mind that for all the similarities, there were also many differences: For example, the first episode occurred in a university medical school hospital in an eastern city, the second in a Church-related community hospital in a large midwestern city. Unquestionably, this circumstance alone accounted for many of the most visible differences. Thus the corridor parade in the teaching hospital was heavily male as squads of surgeon-professors, residents, interns, fellows and clerks danced their roles in the choreography of the nursing floor; the Church hospital, in contrast, was overwhelming female, and the doctors when they did appear were usually unaccompanied.

Unquestionably, too, the varying functions of teaching and Church hospitals accounted for another dissimilarity: As it happened the patient's room in both cases was one nearest the nurses' station—an interesting, if exhausting, listening spot. The conversation in one case was almost exclusively clinical and scientific, punctuated by an occasional note that was social, trivial, scatological, or all three. At the Church hospital, the overheard fragments related mainly to the artifacts of patient care: Did Eight get her enema? Twenty-four scarcely touched her lunch. We ordered the crutches for Seven early this morning and they aren't here yet. I guess we should tell Fifteen that Dr. O called; he won't be in today.

In both instances the patient was a stranger to the institution and its staff, and in both cases he was assigned to a senior staff surgeon—a professor of orthopedics in one case and the head of the department in the other—with a curious result: The professor, a full-time man who by popular stereotype should have been interested in students, not patients, and research, not results, came in at least twice a day, answering questions and offering information and advice in considerable detail, whereas the private practicing surgeon, presumably a devoted worshipper at the altar of the doctor-patient relationship, was glimpsed briefly among the power tools and plaster dust of the cast room, where the rites themselves were carried out by an associate, and then seen once again momentarily a day or two later at the threshold of the patient's room, where he paused long enough to say, "We've ordered you some sticks," and vanished. The associate presided at the discharge, where the instructions consisted wholly of admonitions to (1) keep weight off the leg, (2) be careful, and (3) come back in three weeks.

Now it should be emphasized that there is no suggestion here that the care in the second case was any less skilled, and certainly a part of the difference must be attributed to the fact that the first case was considerably more complex, with more to be done about more fractures. But the contrast was inescapable nevertheless, the more so because the Church hospital staff, or some of its members, are known to be affiliated with the Council of Medical Staffs, an organization whose recruitment efforts lean heavily on the proposition that the A.M.A. isn't doing enough to protect the private practice of medicine and the doctor-patient relationship.

A contrast more likely to have resulted from the difference in time than from the difference in function was the fact that the teaching hospital was virtually all white, whereas the nursing floor at the Church hospital had at least as many black as white faces among the staff. This difference was most noticeable at, but by no means restricted to, the lower levels of skill; there were many R.N.s and technicians, and a sprinkling of physicians, among the non-whites.

As one might expect, too, the difference in time resulted in the fact that the Church hospital had many more visible machines and instruments today than the teaching hospital had 12 years ago—though the most obtrusive instrument, and the noisiest by far in both cases, was the television. For all its machines and noises and traffic of all kinds, however, the Church hospital corridor gave the lesser impression of bustle—a circumstance that owed something to the absence of the dancing doctors, to be sure, but something also, probably, to the fact that the corridor was at least a foot wider. However, the correlation of bustle and confusion was negative: There were two instances of muffed signals at the Church hospital, and none, in a longer stay, at the teaching hospital.

Apparently, time and automation have done nothing to diminish the determination of dietary departments to get patients fed and get out of there, and dinner at 5 o'clock was as inflexible, and at that hour as inedible, in 1972 as it had been in 1960. Also unchanged was the determination of nursing departments to create an archive of temperatures, pulses, respirations and blood pressures of a patient for whom a minimum of these measurements, if any, could have been required for any sensible medical purpose. The record room of the Church hospital, however, remains innocent of any but the barest skeleton of the voluminous medical history that may still bulge the files at the teaching hospital, conceivably having served some purpose or other in the education of an earlier generation of physicians.

Another staple of hospital care, the back rub, remains on the list of compulsory offerings, but here a peculiar variation in hospital practice emerged. At the teaching hospital, the back rub went quickly to the seat of the matter and spent its most energetic efforts at the twin sites that are likely to be troublesome friction points for the supine patient, whereas the back rub at the Church hospital stopped at the equator. There was no way to know, however, whether this represented a difference in delicacy, dedication, philosophy, or knowledge of the etiology of decubitus ulcer; in this as in most other aspects of medical or nursing care, any measurements of quality must comprehend not only the things that are done and not done, but the reasons for the practice, whatever it is.

Only two footnotes need be added to this chronicle: (1) at all levels of skill nurses uniformly fail to comprehend the terrorizing impact of the bedpan, and (2) in the execution of that obscure art form known as the full-leg cast, Harvard leaves less room for the toes than Northwestern does.

Doesn't Anyone Care?

February 1978

"12:10 p.m. Arrived at hospital emergency room," said the report of a Chicago public health nurse, describing her experience with a teenage girl who had come to a city health department clinic in active labor. "Nurse in charge appeared reluctant to accept my description of the patient's status of labor. She asked, 'Did you examine her?' I assured her the clinic physician had examined her. Five or 10 minutes passed before a resident appeared to ask again about the status of the patient. At no time did any hospital employee attempt to monitor patient's contractions, listen for fetal heart tones, or even touch the patient. Finally, the nurse asked me and ambulance attendants to take patient up to labor and delivery department. Patient's contractions were 2 minutes x 50 seconds duration, and she was beginning to experience perineal pressure.

"12.25 p.m. Patient was wheeled to maternity unit, where we were stopped by nurse at front desk. Again I was asked to repeat the same information. We were then told to take the patient into labor and delivery department.

"12:30 p.m. Nurse in labor and delivery again asked me to repeat the same information. I left patient and copies of the clinic record and returned to clinic.

"12:50 p.m. I telephoned hospital labor and delivery unit with some lab reports and was told patient was completely dilated and ready to deliver.

"Later that day I learned she had delivered a stillborn.

"Neither the ambulance attendants nor the hospital personnel demonstrated caring about the patient. It just didn't seem to matter to them. Their tone was not serious and concerned but appeared inappropriate and flippant. The hospital personnel did not attempt to monitor contractions, listen for fetal heart tones, check the perineum, or expedite getting the patient to labor and delivery quickly. I repeated her record and expected delivery date (labor was two months premature) about four times. I think the patient deserved better treatment."

Talking about the episode later, the city nurse said the hospital attitude and behavior at first made her furious, then heartsick as she thought about the young, frightened girl desperately needing sympathetic care and support and receiving instead a kind of treatment it would be considered cruel to give an animal—at a 350-bed, full service, accredited hospital with a reputable medical staff, governing board, and administration. "For all our problems of overload, crowded quarters, and inadequate staff, we provide *care* at the city clinics," she declared.

Assuming that it has been reported accurately, and there is no reason to think otherwise of the report of a nurse with superior professional credentials and obviously humanitarian instincts, the case documents two kinds of error, one that could be expected to evoke prompt and decisive remedial action and another, of greater magnitude, that is more likely to be unremarked, uncorrected, and uncomprehended. The first error was professional inattention, failure to verify the patient's condition and act immediately to prepare for emergency delivery. The receiving nurse, the resident physician, the nurse on the maternity unit, and the one in the labor room all knew better than to sit around asking questions while the patient was in labor. No attending physician, nurse supervisor, or administrator at a hospital of substance would stand for this kind of slipshod professional conduct—not more than once, anyway, and it can be presumed that the culprits have been identified and warned of the consequences of relapse.

The second error is harder to deal with. This was the unfeeling, uncaring attitude that probably resulted in the unprofessional behavior in this case but is nevertheless separate from it, because it often goes hand in hand with what passes for irreproachable professional procedure. The uncaring attitude and the aloof posture that goes along with it are often attributed to simple arrogance, and certainly arrogance is not notably in short supply among physicians and their associates in hospitals. But it seems likely that in more cases than not the causes are a lot more complicated than that. Thus a team of psychiatric investigators a few years ago concluded that the personal remoteness from their patients of emergency department physicians and nurses resulted from repeated and prolonged exposure to professional crisis and emotional stress. "The only way nurses and physicians and other professional people can accommodate the stress is by subconsciously repressing the tendency to become patient oriented," the investigators reported. "Instead, they remain task or profession oriented"—and thus may be seen as uncaring when the fact is they care so much it hurts.

Another cause is that the rise of interest in psychosomatic medicine in our time has by no means arrested, or even seriously modified, the primarily mechanistic approach to medical research and medical practice that had its roots in the dualism of Rene Descartes and has been the prevailing mode of thought in medicine for 300 years. Most physicians today acknowledge the linkage of mind and body, which the Cartesians denied, but the order of importance is evident in the time doctors commonly spend poring over laboratory reports compared to the time spent talking to patients about anything but their symptoms. The Cartesian tradition is giving ground, but slowly. The young physician at the Chicago hospital may have been disciplined for failing to observe the dilation and listen for fetal heart tones, but nobody would think to reprove him because he didn't smile and pat the patient's hand and offer words of encouragement, which may readily have been the more important components of the needed treatment. In fact, it is a rare case in which the spirit doesn't cry out for healing, along with the bones, but it isn't often in today's computerized hospitals that both cries are answered.

Humanists in medicine are inclined to link the absence of caring to the rise of technology, pointing out that it is awkward, if not hazardous, to pat the hands of patients who are wired to machines, and certainly this is part of what has been happening. But the tendency to look at patients as problems rather than persons set in long before most of the machines got there, and, besides, there are notable exceptions demonstrating that it is possible to render tender loving care among the oscillographs. Church hospitals, for example, are often an exception to the trend, and it is an observable phenomenon that the feeling quality of care may vary from floor to floor within the same institution, and even from day to day within the same nursing unit, depending on who's there. This factor can't be measured and fed into the computer—at least not yet—but the sociologists who make a business of patrolling hospital corridors insist that it can be detected if it's present and missed if it isn't.

For the past few years, some medical educators, at least, have been aware that the caring component is more often missed than detected. "Medicine has now become so complicated that in order to be considered competent many physicians feel they must specialize in a narrow area and spend a good part of their time in the laboratory lest their knowledge become dated," Allen R. Dyer, M.D., of Duke University said at the National Congress on Medical Education in 1974. "Tremendous advances have been made in patient care techniques, but patient care nevertheless has suffered." Another lecturer at the same Congress suggested that "the humane physician develops from our medical education system—by chance." Since that time, medical schools increasingly have been emphasizing primary care and reaching out for affiliations with community hospitals, and a growing number of young physicians have been choosing careers in family practice, where, presumably, rewarding personal ties with patients may be established more readily than they can be in the highly specialized medical centers.

These are encouraging developments—but not necessarily for hospitals, where the critical events of the recent past have combined to focus attention on regulation, finance, reimbursement, and planning, to the point where patient care could become again, as it was 50 years ago, something that is left to the doctors to worry about. As it turns out, the doctors who are most inclined to worry about what troubles their patients, as well as what ails them, are likely to be the ones who spend the least time in hospitals. Thus it was that Granger Westberg, D.D., a clergyman who spent 25 years as a hospital chaplain and trainer of hospital chaplains, left the hospital a few years ago to establish the wholistic health centers now operating in a dozen sites in the Midwest and in process of being organized elsewhere. The wholistic centers combine primary medical and nursing care with personal and family counseling aimed at disclosing and dealing with the underlying life circumstances causing stress related to illness. Westberg had become convinced that the hospital was not an effective setting for the exercise of this dimension of care. "We were seen as needed only when the doctors had given up," he said. Politely, Dr. Westberg attributed the absence of caring to lack of time, not lack of interest, and unquestionably time pressures are a part of the problem.

It doesn't have to be that way. Where the wholistic health centers seek to add a new element of caring that is provided outside the hospital by trained counselors and volunteers, another experimental approach to caring, the Institute for the Study of Humanistic Medicine in San Francisco, is exploring another route to the same goal. The Institute is training physicians and nurses to bring their scientific and technologic processes to bear on the human needs of people, comprehending the mind, the body, the will, and the aspirations. The Institute is committed to the proposition that physicians, nurses, and others can be compassionate as well as competent, Dale C. Garrell, M.D., medical director, explained, listing the principles it is teaching as (1) the patient must not be seen simply as his disease; (2) health is the dynamic integration of body, mind, emotion, and spirit; (3) the patient and the physician are colleagues in the health relationship, and (4) illness must be seen in the context of the life span of the individual, not 15 minutes or two months. "The goal is to overcome the tendency of the scientific and technologic processes of medicine to dehumanize medical care." Garrell said.

It shouldn't take a whole new approach to medical education and medical care in order to humanize the processes of medicine. By anybody's definition, it is poor medicine to mend the bodily system and leave the troubled spirit unheeded, and poorer still to mend the system and hurt the spirit in the process. Forgetting that the system and the spirit are one inseparable person is not a product of technology, and it is not new. "It seems to some of us who hear the recitals of poor people after they come back from the hospital as if the patient were not the chief concern," said Jane Addams, the celebrated humanitarian who was the founder of Chicago's Hull House settlement, in an address to a group of physicians and hospital superintendents in Chicago 50 years ago. She told about a patient in need of attention who had watched as a nearby nurse kept on folding and refolding sheets. "I suppose it is very important to have sheets folded in a certain way and present a better appearance to the visiting staff," Miss Addams said. "It is true, perhaps, that some things in hospital wards have been exalted into a kind of institutional test, and no one stops to inquire whether it has been made tidy at the expense of the comfort of some patient. Somehow or other the machine goes on. It lacks adaptation. It lacks power of readjustment. It does not quite rise to the occasion. If it is the business of the hospital to treat diseases as such, to treat them so that the hospital will have a splendid record and put down so many cases as cured, then this indictment is quite unfair and I apologize for it. If perchance it should be the more humane aim to care for those members of society and to send them back so that they may take up the work of life again, then it seems to me the hospitals are open to some measure of indictment."

So they were then, and so they still are, and all it really takes to make the indictment quite unfair is dedication to the more humane aim to care for those members of society so that they may take up the work of life again. Everybody knows how.

If We Don't Care,
They Won't

October 1978

A few weeks ago, I spent a day or two at a mountain resort with the board of trustees of a community hospital, at one of those occasions that have come to be known—somewhat infelicitously, it has seemed to me—as retreats. At one point in the program, the board had scheduled a discussion of internal business affairs and asked me to meet at that time with the husbands and wives of board members and talk with them about their community relations responsibilities, an assignment that was vague enough to suggest that it was essentially a polite way of getting us all out from underfoot at the business meeting.

The hospital was one of two good, and good sized, institutions in the community, which was still small enough so it seemed likely that most of the neighbors, friends, and acquaintances of the husbands and wives would know they were connected with the hospital in some way, but not so closely, as physicians, nurses, administrators, and trustees themselves are, that people would be reluctant to let them know what their real feelings about the hospital were, for reasons that are sugggested by the old Hindu proverb: "Before thou fordest the river, O Brother, revile not unduly the crocodile's mother." So I started by asking the group to tell me what kinds of things they heard about the hospital. What do people say to you about their hospital experiences? I asked. What do they complain about? What do they ask you? What do they tell you they hear other people say?

As it turned out, the first thing that was mentioned was a complaint about delay and confusion in the emergency department, and it developed that just about everybody had heard something about emergency services—mostly delays, and mostly having to do with things that doctors wouldn't consider real emergencies. But something else needs to be reported here first, and that is the fact that this conversation on the way

175

people feel about hospitals went on for more than an hour before anybody mentioned cost, and when it did come up the complaint was not that the cost was too high but that people couldn't understand their hospital bills or their insurance coverage and had a hard time getting anybody to explain them so they could be understood. The things these wives and husbands of trustees reported being said about the hospital rarely had to do with the substantive content of medical care, either. The way things are today, apparently, those who aren't satisfied with their medical care don't talk about it. They just sue.

The complaints and worries, in this community as in most others, are concerned for the most part with things physicians and hospital administrators and trustees consider unimportant—waiting time in emergency departments, outpatient departments, diagnostic departments, nursing floors, all over. As we talked about these things in some detail, it was agreed that what bothers patients and families isn't just that there are delays and waits; everybody understands that in complex schedules and services there are bound to be delays. The thing that irritates and upsets people is *unexplained* delay and waiting. It isn't the confusion of requests for information or the things that have to be done during admission and on the floors, it's the fact that nobody has explained what is going on or why the information is needed. In this discussion with the wives and husbands and in many others that I've had with people about their hospital experiences, in all kinds of hospitals in all parts of the country, phrases that I've heard over and over again are: Nobody bothered. Nobody took the trouble. Nobody seemed to care. Nobody told me. Nobody explained. And, often, "I didn't dare ask." The endless details of admission and discharge, the repetitive questions, the long waits can all be endured. The not knowing what's going on is frightening. But the indifference or aloofness, or sometimes downright rudeness, is infuriating.

How could we have gotten to a point where the patients we are concerned about, and care about, and are caring for, and trying to help, can possibly say a thing like "I didn't dare ask"—with all that it implies about the attitudes they are confronted with in their hospital experiences? I think there are probably several reasons that need examining, but it is only fair to point out first that indifference, aloofness, and rudeness are not encountered only in hospital offices, rooms, and corridors; they are rampant throughout the society. We complain all the time about surliness in stores and offices; teachers denounce the conduct of students and students that of teachers; businessmen couldn't care less about pleasing their customers. Ask a bus driver a question—and run for your life.

Why? One reason is that we move about so much now that we're all strangers to one another. There are still families that have lived in the same communities for generations, but there are more than ever before who change houses and streets and towns as easily as they change clothes, and this changes the way they relate to neighbors and businesses and schools and churches, and certainly to doctors and hospitals. Another reason is that we know more. More of us have been to school for more years than was the case with our parents. They were inclined to take things as they came, but we want things better, and quicker. Demanding behavior evokes efficiency on occasion, but it also evokes the peremptory response; the reply churlish calls for the countercheck quarrelsome.

Most significantly, however, it is the technology that is changing everything. We are fed, housed, moved, taught, steered, and bullied by machines, and many of us relate to machines for more hours than we do to human beings. The sociologists who tell us how much television has changed our lives and our value system frequently mention its impact in the family and in the classroom, but the President's Commission on Medical Malpractice a few years ago also found that the doctor shows and the medical commercials have elevated the public expectation of medicine unrealistically, to the point where the absence of miracles is often regarded as a cause for action. With patients like that, only saints can be patient.

Television chases us into the hospital when we are sick, to be sure, but here the tube is outnumbered and outfaced by the oscillograph. The machines on the floors are formidable, but the machines in the diagnostic departments are positively intimidating. Patients may be cowed by machines, but doctors and nurses are ruled by them. Patients and families ask dumb questions; computers and oscillographs give stern orders. The moving needle writes, and having writ, moves on; nor all your dignity nor wit shall lure it back to cancel half a line. The machine makes patients jumpy, but it makes doctors jump. "As medical technology increases, it increases the psychological distance between doctor and patient and the imposed passivity of the patient," a contemporary observer says. "As the doctor retreats further into his scientific cocoon, his words and actions become less and less comprehensible to the patient, while at the same time the patient's words and actions become less and less important to the doctor's diagnosis and treatment of the condition. Taking a history and performing a physical examination, which classically have been the basis of medical diagnosis and which require direct doctor-patient contact and the active cooperation of the patient, have steadily declined in importance relative to a growing array of diagnostic procedures that develop detached, objectified evidence of pathology. These typically involve the patient only in the minimal, passive contact of offering his body up to nurses and technicians while they extract from it blood, X-ray pictures, or squiggles on a graph."[1]

The same observer describes what has been happening to our doctors: "The fact that research dollars flowed to investigators located at medical schools meant that medical school faculties came increasingly to comprise physicians who were scientific researchers as much as, if not more than, they were practitioners of medicine. The role models then presented to successive waves of medical students came increasingly to be people who saw and projected themselves as scientists more than as healers . . . The biomedical model and the ideology of excellence thus inevitably downgrade the interpersonal aspects of the encounter between patient and doctor or hospital worker, such considerations being shrugged off as unscientific." You don't dare ask questions of a biomedical model.

Sixty years after the creation of the Hospital Standardization Program of the American College of Surgeons, it is possible finally to consider that there are standards by which, within limits, the scientific and technical content of the quality of medical care may be measured, and this is being done right along. But there are still no standards for measuring the effectiveness of the doctor-patient relationship, or patient satisfaction, or physician satisfaction, although these might also be considered important components of quality, along with continuity of care, patient education, and the behavior of nurses, technicians, and others who take part in the processes of patient care. "Performance measures of quality should give significant weight to customer satisfaction," John R. Griffith of the University of Michigan Bureau of Hospital Administration, said. "It is important to recognize that quality measures must reflect both the curing and the caring aspects of service. While the patient and his family may be easily misled about the technical services of hospitals, they are the best, and possibly the only, judges of care in its most fundamental definition—whether the hospital personnel were humane, sensitive and responsive. Much of the service provided by hospitals is not for cure but for relief of pain, anxiety, and disability. No way has yet been found to quantify these elements on a discharge abstract, yet their importance is much too great to overlook. Consumers sometimes seem to put more emphasis on these factors and others like convenience, kindness, friendliness, amenities, and comfort than they do on more measurable and technical quality elements."[2]

Griffith is convinced that a carefully designed and administered post-discharge sample survey of patients would produce valid and reliable data to measure these components of quality, and he has obtained support for a research project aimed at developing and testing an instrument for producing the data. Meanwhile, it would appear that there are some things every hospital could do to improve performance in these aspects of quality, assuming some agreement that these *are* aspects of quality. The first would be to make an assessment of existing practice and performance, not by the usual perfunctory patient opinion polls that never reflect anything more than the crocodile effect, but by carefully planned interviews conducted by trained interviewers away from the hospital, and by objective observations of the way hospital people behave at the critical points such as outpatient and emergency departments, admission and discharge, diagnostic departments, and nursing floors. It seems likely that if these inquiries and investigations don't disclose any lapses from acceptable behavior toward patients, families, and visitors, the hospital would have to be either blessed or blind.

Experienced administrators don't need to be told how to go about improving performance where this is seen as needed and desirable. As with any other aspect of hospital operations, the method includes defining the problem, seeking the causes, establishing the specific objectives for change, making plans with executives, department heads, and supervisors, and evaluating the results. As always, too, finding out what others are doing, or have done, and with what results, is part of the process. Some hospitals have hired consultants to conduct training sessions for sensitive personnel; others have recruited and trained ombudsmen, patient representatives, or specialists in patient education. Some have used hospital chaplains to assist with the effort, and some use volunteers.

Certainly a part of the program, and perhaps the most important part, would have to be initiated and conducted by and for members of the medical staff. Nurses and aides and technicians who observe physicians giving patients and visitors the brush-off are not exactly inspired to take pains to be friendly and responsive in their own behavior, or to be persuaded that it really matters whether they are or not. But on every staff there are some physicians who care and can set an example, and probably many who are unaware that their behavior could ever be anything but exemplary and need only to be reminded by caring colleagues that how they look and act and speak establishes the emotional tone that can either comfort or destroy the spirit. For all the influence of the academic-scientific biomedical model, there can't be many doctors of medicine who really don't give a damn for their patients.

If administrators and trustees and a few physicians think it's important, they'll think of many more ways to improve the quality of caring in their hospitals. There may even be some who think, as I do, that a great, organized, national voluntary effort to improve the quality of caring could be at least as important to the future of our hospital system as the great, organized, national voluntary cost containment effort is. If I am wrong, and if administrators and trustees and doctors, or many of them, consider that it doesn't really matter, or that "I didn't dare ask" is the right attitude to inculcate in patients and families and visitors, because they're a lot less trouble that way, then none of these things are going to be done to change the way people are regarded and treated in hospitals. In that case, patients and families and communities probably won't care very much whether our hospitals survive as free institutions or whether they become just another so-called public service like the post office and the license bureau and the city hall, because they won't be able to tell the difference.

[1]Lander, L., Defective Medicine: Risk, Anger and the Malpractice Crisis, New York: Farrar, Straus & Giroux, 1978.

[2]Griffith, J.R., Measuring Hospital Performance, Chicago: Blue Cross Association, 1978.

The PR War Isn't
the Real War

August 1979

Speaking on the voluntary cost containment effort at an American Medical Association leadership conference, Michael Bromberg of the Federation of American Hospitals said, "We're losing the public relations war. We're not getting our message over, and people are being persuaded that with mandatory controls they can have national health insurance at no added cost. We've got to answer this."

Without diminishing either the gravity of the cost containment problem or the need to use every means to avoid mandatory controls, it is possible to raise questions about these assumptions. While it is apparent that hospitals and doctors are losing the competition for headlines and television news time, if that's what is meant by the public relations war, it is not by any means certain that public opinion goes with the headlines. And while people have been told the mandatory controls on hospitals are prerequisite to national health insurance, there isn't much evidence either that they believe it or that they care very much one way or the other. In this as in other matters we have a tendency to assume that everybody else is as interested in health affairs as we are, but we ought to know better; except for those who are sick, many other things come first—family, jobs, money, housing, food, clothes, cars, gasoline, vacation, and entertainment, to name a few. These are everyday, particular experiences with which the hospital can compete for attention only as it becomes immediate and particular.

That's what it is for patients and their families, and that's what it may become for others under some special circumstances, such as when the hospital becomes a place of refuge for many in cases of disaster. Sometimes the disaster is threatened rather than actual, and if the threat is seen as immediate and particular, public opinion may emerge from its accustomed preoccupations and make itself evident with astonishing force. This is what happened, for example, when the health planning guidelines were first published in September 1977 and some communities discovered that their hospitals would be cut down, and possibly shut down, if the guidelines were to become enforceable rules. In the first few weeks following publication of the guidelines, the Health Resources Administration in HEW got 55,000 letters of protest, and the number reportedly reached 70,000 before the controversy subsided. Along the way, HRA got interested enough to analyze the returns and find out what happened. As it turned out, the analysis focused on Iowa and Texas; more than half the letters came from these two states. HRA staff and a consultant reviewed these and selected two communities whose letters seemed personal and responsive rather than perfunctory or canned, and came from people who weren't associated with hospitals. In July 1978, the consultant visited Sibley, IA, and New Braunfels, TX, and interviewed 40 or 50 people in each case to find out what had prompted such an outpouring of public opinion.

The first thing he found out was that the response was spontaneous. "Local citizens initiated the letter-writing campaigns in both communities," the consultant said. "Although the Iowa and Texas hospital and medical societies actively opposed the guidelines, the response in Sibley and New Braunfels was entirely local. There was no participation by an organization or interest outside the community."[1] In both cases, too, it was the guideline that would have required 500 births a year to keep an obstetric department open that had touched off the fireworks. The 80 percent occupancy requirement also threatened both hospitals, but the primary fear had been that young mothers would have to leave their families and leave town to have their babies.

The indignation was intensified by the fact that the standard was imposed by federal authority. "The guidelines hit a raw nerve in this community," a New Braunfels hospital trustee told the consultant. "Here were some bureaucrats in Washington sitting in an ivory tower telling people they can no longer bring their children into this world in their own community. Here was someone who probably doesn't know where New Braunfels is telling the people of New Braunfels where to have their babies." In both towns there were hair-raising stories of women who wouldn't have made it to a hospital 40 or 50 miles away. "I delivered my last one in 22 minutes, and that wouldn't even be time to get to the highway," a Texas mother said, and a minister who had urged his parishioners to write letters recounted the sudden delivery of a son born with breathing difficulty requiring special attention. "If we had been forced to drive to San Antonio, it is likely that because of the distance our son would have been born en route and, because of the difficulties, would have died," he said.

Other stories had to do with emergency injuries and sudden illnesses. "Almost everyone interviewed in Sibley had a story of someone who would not be with us or would have been permanently maimed or harmed if the hospital did not exist," the report said. "These accounts focused on people who had suffered heart attacks, children involved in accidents or becoming ill, persons injured while working on their farms or at their jobs. In addition, the residents mentioned the hardships that would be imposed on families that had to travel that far to visit someone in the hospital, as well as the expense and disruption of family life that would occur." People over 65 were especially troubled by the prospect of losing the hospital. "I don't know what we would do if my husband or I became sick and the hospital wasn't here. It scares me," said an elderly resident of Sibley, where 20 percent of the population is over age 65.

The fear was caused by the anticipated loss of service, but the fury that helped to spark the response arose from the way the threat came about. These were some of the comments:

"I'm on the state education board, and I've had enough experience to know that guidelines often have the effect of law."

"They were not goals. They are actually rules. They were going to take the hospital out of our community."

"These so-called nonenforceable things become enforced."

"Technically, they can't make you meet the guidelines if you don't want to. But they can cut your money off and make you sorry you didn't."

"If they didn't think they would enforce them in the future, then why did they draw them up?"

"You are an ostrich with your head stuck in the sand if you believe they're not enforceable. I can't see them spending all that time on something that couldn't be enforced."

"I felt they were mandatory. The intimidation was there. The attitude was: If you don't believe us, just wait and see."

Months after the guidelines were modified and the pressure relieved, there was still a residue of mistrust. "I'm still not sure where we stand," a Sibley man said. "We won the battle but the war is still going on. I wouldn't bet on this hospital being open 10 years from now." And in New Braunfels the hospital administrator warned, "The revisions are not letting us off the hook." Moreover, most of the people didn't feel that HEW had revised the guidelines because they had written the letters. The people of Sibley felt they had been effective chiefly because they had also written their representative and senator. "As more than one person pointed out, HEW can afford to ignore 1,000 or 2,000 letters from northwest Iowa, but Berkley Bedell and Dick Clark cannot afford that luxury," the report said. "The federal government responded to political pressures."

However it came about, there can't be much question that this was an occasion when public opinion was on the side of the hospitals and said so, fortissimo—something that doesn't happen every day. Probably it couldn't have happened this way in a large metropolitan area, but there are instances even here of latent feeling evoked by particular experience, as when people walked in off the street to see if they could help New York hospitals crippled by the celebrated 1965 power failure. The rule seems plain enough: Abstractions like regulation and government and cost containment and national health insurance awake only a flicker of interest, and even less response, but when the focus is immediate and particular, the abstraction we call the public becomes a critical mass of men and women who know what they want and say so, in what may be a living demonstration of a proposition that has been around ever since the 14th century, when William of Occam's Law of Parsimony, or "Occam's razor," postulated that only particular things are real. Classes or concepts of things are only names, Occam insisted. It was an argument that made the Scholastic philosophers and theologians of his time nervous, and it may make our leaders and officials and consultants nervous today to consider that the concepts and policies they worry about are only names and are going to be largely ignored by all the rest of us unless or until they become real experiences.

There ought to be a public relations lesson here. The headlines and news broadcasts we long to see and hear reporting the great work hospitals are doing would be forgotten as quickly as the headlines about hospital waste and inefficiency and unnecessary surgery are, by everybody except the few whose particular experience is immediately affected. This suggests that a large part of the public relations effort should be directed not so much toward creating or defending against headlines as toward making as certain as it can be done that the hospital's work *is* great and the waste and inefficiency and unnecessary surgery are eliminated. As it commonly is in industry today, the public relations function in hospitals thus needs to be elevated to the top level of policymaking and management, not left in the hands of us communications technicians.

Now a lot of public opinion experts think that lasting and important impressions, or images, as they like to call them, are created by what people read in newspapers and magazines and what they see on television. A man in my business can't afford to get caught saying that what people read in newspapers and magazines makes no difference at all in what they think, so I shall acknowledge that people may indeed be impressed by what they read, perhaps even to the point of forming fleeting opinions, but only if they have no particular experience of the subject, or if what they read confirms their experience. If what they read contradicts what they know at first hand, the knowledge or feeling is not likely to be wiped out by the impression of the printed page or the tube.

Nevertheless, articles and lectures and discussions on the hospital image abound. The point of many of these exercises is that the hospital image is something different from, and worse than, the hospital itself, that the image in some way can be manipulated and improved, that this had better be done right away, and that when it is done many, if not most, of the problems of public understanding and public support and public policy will vanish. This kind of image worry and image worship, it should be noted, is endemic in the society. Business, for example, is at least as obsessed with concern about its image as hospitals are with theirs. Labor, government, the professions, and even the Church share the same belief that what they are and what they do are perfectly all right, actually, but the public has got them all wrong somehow and needs straightening out. But in the case of hospitals it seems likely that the thing that needs straightening out is not so much the image as the mistaken notion that it is bad or that it could ever be anything very different from the experience. Opinion polls consistently reporting 80 or 90 percent of people well satisfied with hospital care suggest that the experience is good, and that people everywhere would respond to the threat of curtailment or suspension of their hospital services the way the people of Sibley and New Braunfels did. But the threat has to be as immediate and particular as $1 bread or $2 gas. It isn't that real yet, and we won't find out if we've won or lost the public opinion war until the war is over.

[1]Danaceau, P., The Health Planning Guidelines Controversy: A Report from Iowa and Texas. Washington, DC: Office of Planning, Evaluation and Legislation, Health Resources Administration, U.S. Dept. of Health, Education, and Welfare, Reprinted by the Iowa Hospital Association, January 1979.

What You See Can Help
Shape What You Get

June 1980

The public perception of a health care institution may owe something to identity or name recognition, but unless these are solidly based on real values of excellent performance and caring service, recognition will be empty of meaning, like the brightly wrapped packages in a Christmas store-window display. But it doesn't follow that identity or image is only wrapping; it has intrinsic worth as well, because the use of service it promotes and the sense of community it evokes help the institution move toward its goals. And neither competent service nor compassionate care nor effective communication of these values can be accomplished unless the institution's management, physicians, and personnel are aware of the identity, the services, and the goals. The image can never be exactly the same outside as it is inside, but disharmonies in the boardroom or the doctor's lounge or the employees' cafeteria will damage community perceptions over time by subtracting something from performance. Thus the image and the values it reflects must emerge from unchanging principles of right action that inform an institutional mission whose goals are always clearly visible.

This view of public or community relations as an essential component of the hard bones and long muscles of the institutional corpus, and not just its outer skin, emerged from a full day of deep thinking and spirited talk by some 30 members of the executive staff of the Catherine McAuley Health Center (CMHC) at Ann Arbor, MI—one of a series of such exercises initiated following creation of the center as a division of the Sisters of Mercy Health Corp. Others discussions were focused on program objectives; the session on identity was occasioned when the new Catherine McAuley Health Center took over the operation of two existing hospitals and it became apparent that some people inside the institutions, and most people outside, were asking, "What's this?"

One thing that it is became clear as soon as it developed that there were one or two members of the discussion group who weren't sure themselves about the answer: The Catherine McAuley Health Center is an accomplished fact. It isn't going to go away or be subordinated to any of its constituent parts. It was created to provide an appropriate entity for development of a comprehensive, integrated system of health services for the community, beginning with the existing acute general hospital and psychiatric hospital, already expanded to include a neighborhood outpatient clinic, and starting now to investigate needs and formulate plans for services to the elderly. There were misgivings that the name "center" had a geographic connotation that might prove to be confusing, if not misleading, for a corporate entity having widely dispersed parts, and it was suggested that "services" or "system" might be preferable under the circumstances. In fact, one small discussion group recommended that "services" should be substituted for "center" in the corporate name but there was no broad consensus that this should be done, and it seemed likely that the center would remain a center.

Plainly it wouldn't be easy, and there were some who thought it wouldn't be possible. But there weren't as many of those at the end of the day as there had been at the beginning, in part because of the many suggestions for making the positive values of institutional services felt inside and outside the organization, and in part also because a consultant to the group throughout the day had emphasized the importance of moral principles underlying the services, and there had been no doubts about the moral righteousness of institutions founded and dedicated to "bring mercy and compassion to those in need, reach out to those suffering from illness, and render public witness to Christ's love for all persons."

The consultant was Carl Cohen, Ph.D., professor of philosophy at the University of Michigan, and he had warned at the outset that the principles were subject to strain. "There is, I think, in the world of health care provision a tendency, especially in these latter days, to weigh efficiency too heavily, in the occasional collision between efficiency and equity to give considerations of fairness not quite enough weight," he said. But after listening and taking part in the group's deliberations, Cohen had seemed confident that it would come out on the right side of the efficiency *vs.* equity struggle that is a central tension within the health care culture today. "The concern for moral principle is very clearly embedded in the history of the Sisters of Mercy order and the work of Catherine McAuley (founder of the order)," he said in a concluding comment, "and all of that remains reverberating in the thinking of these discussion groups as they met. It deserves to be treasured, and it is one of the great strengths of the Catherine McAuley Health Center and of its elements, much to be prized."

As a philosopher with a tilt toward utilitarianism, Cohen went on to point out that principles were not to be considered altogether apart from programs. "Intellect can and should be put to the service of morality," he said. "In advancing the values that we prize, we can think very carefully about competing ways of doing it, competing paths that are open to us, and we can put reason to our service in all of this."

A difficulty that kept getting in the way of making selections from among competing paths or activities was that reason seemed to come down on both sides of two sets of choices of ways to go in seeking identity or recognition for the Catherine McAuley Health Center: the choice between pushing the center with possible loss to the established identities of the existing hospitals, or clinging to the hospital names and hoping the "What's this?" question would eventually go away; and the choice between emphasizing comprehensive services yet to be established, at the possible risk of allowing the image to outrun the substance, or holding back until the services were in place. Arguing on the "go slow" side of both choices, another consultant to the group had said, "You shouldn't ever undervalue the names that are already familiar to the constituency you're going to be dealing with. These are feelings and attitudes based on a particular experience, and I don't think you can ever wholly explain the added services that you intend to provide to the community in order to secure their better health care until these services do·become particular experiences."

As it turned out, the prevailing view was that it wasn't really that big a problem. Somebody mentioned how quickly Esso had given way to Exxon. A design consultant demonstrated how corporations speedily and successfully achieve recognition of their changing structures and components through planned use of identifying symbols and advertising. He suggested several variations of usage that the group agreed could help capture the desired recognition of Catherine McAuley and still retain all the values—for the hospital personnel, the medical staff, and the community—in the established good names of St. Joseph Mercy and Mercywood hospitals. But the most persuasive reasoning was that "by communicating what we wish to become, we can in fact facilitate our becoming the Catherine McAuley Health Center and reaching our full potential." That was the considered opinion of CMHC president Robert Laverty, for whom the full potential meant not just the envisioned comprehensive services but also a leadership role in community thought.

"You have an opportunity to examine a range of issues in a very comprehensive way," Laverty told the group, "and there may be a responsibility to influence the community, not in the sense of propaganda but by taking a position of wanting the community to know what are some of the critical health issues we face—not necessarily taking a position on those issues as much as presenting the different points of view in a scholarly way. Why shouldn't the Catherine McAuley Health Center be looked at as a resource, at least in this community, of some clear thinking on what some of the critical issues are that the community faces, and the way to address those issues?"

The Laverty concept was discussed at length in one of the small groups, where there was agreement that "we wanted to be an organization that was willing to take risks based on a commitment to the individual and the community, a kind of intellectual base that moves the community ahead with demands for development. First of all, we wanted to instill in all of us, as employees or people connected with the organization, that sense of tradition, that sense of values, and then to take action based on some kind of thoughtful response to issues, and not just open for business every day."

As there began to emerge from that kind of talk the feeling that the Catherine McAuley Health Center could become something more than the sum of its parts, something special that might attend not only the needs for medical care and emotional and spiritual comfort of its patients and their families but in some ways also the spirit or vital principle of a whole community, it became apparent that the place to begin was at home. And there was work to be done here. As is the case more often than not in mergers and corporate maneuvers of all kinds, employees—or many of them—felt left out. It wasn't, and isn't ever, that nobody had thought to tell them what was going on, so much as simply that nobody knew just what to say. Publications for employees had said as much as could be told, but there hadn't been time or information enough to permit the kind of detailed, face-to-face communication with department heads, supervisors, and employee groups that gets all the questions out and answered. It would take a series of such meetings, over time, to "instill in all of us that sense of values," that the discussants had seen as needed. "We felt that there has not been much discussion with the employees and medical staff of the different units in terms of what the Catherine McAuley Health Center was and what should be done," the leader of another small group said in his report.

Inevitably, there was talk of audiences, and understanding that there would have to be different emphases, and different methods of communication, for different groups. One discussion session listed 37 separate audiences for which information should be provided. Another listed almost as many separate messages to be communicated, still another the media or methods of transmission necessarily involved. And at the concluding meeting Richard Price, Ph.D., professor and chairman of the department of community psychology at the University of Michigan and also a consultant to CMHC, spoke of what remained to be done. "You've spent the last two hours talking about critical publics, program initiatives, goals or expectations, and values," he said. "Some hard intellectual work needs to be done now to put those four things together. They need to be cross-hatched. You need to ask how they match up. Whatever next steps you take ought to produce an output or a product down the line, and then it seems to me you need to take another cut at this. And in fact it needs to be an iterative, repetitive, recycling process."

Earlier, Price had presented an analysis of how knowledge and attitudes are communicated, or, in psychologists' terms, "how the natural social environments of community members interact with the service environments of hospitals and other human service organizations. It's really the coming together of two worlds, and how they come together, how carefully they're designed to mesh with one another, is a critical issue in thinking about what your image is, what your identity is, how you relate to the community." Information and attitudes are shaped to a large extent by the primary groups or social networks of which we are all members, Price explained, our families, friends, neighbors, work associates, and others who are part of our daily lives and have a powerful influence on our standards, our values, and our behavior. "The prevailing attitudes and norms in those smaller worlds or networks play a large role in deciding which paths people take when they're considering the use of professional help," he added.

Networks have varying compositions with varying qualities and characteristics, Price suggested, and illustrating the point by a simple sociogram on the blackboard, he explained how persons he identified as "boundary spanners" with ties to more than one group may link these and transmit information, attitudes, and behavior within the larger community. This happens most frequently in relatively diffuse networks whose members are joined by only a few links, as in common occupations, and only rarely in "dense" groups sharing ethnic or neighborhood ties, where everybody knows everybody else. "Weak ties can be critical sources of new information, while strong ties in a network tend to recirculate old information," Price said, giving definition to a familiar phenomenon. "This is sometimes called the strength of weak ties, and it's an important thing to understand about the structure of social networks and how they transmit information."

During the meeting, an observer had noted recommendation for firming up the name and deciding on the manner of its presentation in varying contexts; preserving a favorable balance of equity and efficiency; promoting the values as well as the services, and the plans as well as the performance; taking public positions on issues as leaders of community thought should do; programming face-to-face communication and open discussion with members of the medical staff and employees; undertaking the painstaking task of matching up lists of publics, initiatives, goals, and values, and establishing a procedure for keeping the match-ups current; identifying and taking the temperatures of the community's social networks and boundary spanners as the data base for designing services and imprinting institutional values on the community; and formulating a strategy for use of all the available media to advance institutional purposes.

Bringing these objectives to life in working policies and programs would obviously involve not just the community relations staff that was seeking guidance from the group, but the whole organization and all its parts. At a time when specialization of function makes all organizations increasingly complex, and professional institutions, especially, have a tendency to become loose federations of professions and support services with diverse interests and objectives, as opposed to coherent organisms, the identity project thus offered a rare opportunity to benefit from the unifying effects of common purpose and shared activity. To capture the benefits, the organization would need to remember Cohen's emphasis on underlying principle and his warning about the threatening ascendancy of efficiency over equity in a technological era. He had also cautioned against seeking simplicity at the expense of accuracy, another temptation in an age of complexity, with special relevance for communications. "Clear, simple messages will never do the job of explicating the manifold functions of the Catherine McAuley Health Center," he said. "Whatever it is that turns out to guide us will not be simple. There will be a tendency to slip into slogans and rely on catchwords when what will be needed will be much more lengthy refinement of judgment and analysis of principle." Referring to Aristotle's metaphor in the *Rhetoric* of a man passing an observer so swiftly that his features are indistinguishable, he advised care lest the drive for clarity, vividness and impact should invade accuracy. "I do urge refinement of statement, analysis of competing claims, careful justification of policies, with principles made explicit. It's going to be complicated, and the consequence is going to be that we are not going to be understood by portions of our publics who will not have the patience or perhaps even the capacity to understand the refinements. But even at the cost of delayed understanding or partial misunderstanding, choose complexity over excessive simplicity, for the sake of accuracy and precision in the long run. The reputation and the character of the Catherine McAuley Health Center will grow as the honesty and accuracy of its account of itself come to be respected."

Finally, Cohen counseled, give process breathing room in its inevitable conflicts with substance. "In our administrative roles, or as a committee, or whatever, we may know the solution to a given problem," he said. "But we may know also that there is a right process by which that decision should be made. And it may happen that the right process will reach a result which we understand to be mistaken. This is all too common a circumstance in the operation of complex organizations. But it's terribly important, it seems to me, that we should respect a just and rational process in the resolution of the issues that will be before us. The appropriate processes will differ greatly, depending on the issues. In fact, a great deal of decision making in the world of health care provision is and ought to be hierarchical; there is and ought to be an appropriate chain of command of responsibility and obedience. But also a good deal of important decision making is democratic and involves the process of equal participation by a body of equals who, as a body, are charged with the responsibility for a particular task. What happens, then, when a conflict arises and a properly charged, properly deliberative, and properly thoughful body nevertheless comes to a result which you and I know is wrong?

"Of course, doing the right thing is what it's all about. Substance is what counts. But we also want right action not only on this question but on questions like this, over a chain of time. Therefore I suggest cautiously that when our organs are fundamentally healthy, as I have every reason to suppose they are and will be, we should respect their processes. Three prudential considerations support this suggestion: First, we are likely to get the best sum of results if we stick with procedural rules that we are confident are just; if we scrap the rules to get a particular result we know to be desirable, our chain of results over time is likely to be not so good. Secondly, if our process is a decent one, it's going to allow for a certain amount of self-correction, and we should have confidence in ourselves, our subordinates, and our ability to self-correct. And third—the hardest perhaps to swallow—knowing that X is what ought to be done but Y is what they decided to do, we may be wrong. There may be a wisdom that we did not see, and the only hope to find such wisdoms as we may have missed is by respecting good process. Let us therefore be substance-oriented but process-minded."

An organization that can live by these precepts will not be long finding the identity it seeks.

Getting the Message
Where It Counts

April 1980

In a book called *The Powers That Be,* David Halberstam examined the history, organizational structure, current operations, and influence of CBS, Time, Inc., The Washington Post Co., and the Los Angeles Times-Mirror Co., which he considers to be the most powerful communications networks influencing public opinion in America today. He left out the *New York Times* and its subsidiary periodical and book-publishing enterprises because the *Times* had been thoroughly dissected in a book by Gay Talese a few years ago. The Halberstam book, in addition to being a fascinating account of the inner workings and personalities of the media giants, is also a thoughtful analysis of how the communications technology and the minds that direct its applications affect values in the society, and especially how they have become dominant factors in how we think about political issues and how we evaluate political candidates. In fact, according to Halberstam, television has made the two-party system as it has worked for generations in American politics virtually inoperative in our time.

But no example of Halberstam's was as dramatically revealing as the one that unfolded during the winter just past as the political crises in Iran and Afghanistan took over the headlines and news broadcasts. While the actual situations seemed to remain essentially unchanged for weeks at a time, because of the worldwide implications of what was happening the media were obliged to keep reporting day by day; to make certain of having something other than another day of suspense to report, they sought out public officials in Teheran and Washington and elsewhere and extracted statements that were printed and broadcast and may thus have had a bearing on what happened. The effect inevitably was multiplied as newspapers and TV networks competed for the most compelling stories—going so far, it was alleged, as to encourage or even stage-manage some of the hostile demonstrations that made the most shocking pictures. The pictures in turn had their own consequences, though whether or not they could have had any substantive effect on what happened will probably never be known.

What is known is that the events, real and surreal, have already had some effect on presidential politics in the United States as the candidates maneuver for preference and position in the volatile public opinion polls, whose scores are scrutinized jealously by the political masterminds. The polls themselves are thought to have an influence on how people vote, the theory apparently being that the voters care more about backing a winner than they do about who wins. Either way, poll results may dictate where the candidates go and what they say when they get there—a process that isn't exactly what members of the Constitutional Convention had in mind when they spelled out the method for selecting someone to be Commander in Chief of the Army and Navy, make treaties, and from time to time give the Congress information on the State of the Union.

However painful the events themselves may be to contemplate, the putative war in the Middle East and the preoccupation with presidential candidate antics have diverted the public opinion polls, and the resulting headlines, away from the horrors of health care costs that were a staple of the news business most of last year. But this is more reprieve than pardon; the pressure on costs is unrelenting, and the headlines will be back whenever one of the polls wants to take a breather from the candidate count and can think of another way to ask the health care cost question in a fashion that seems certain to evoke answers that will cause gasps. In a circular manner not unlike the demonstrations that beget headlines that beget reprisals that beget demonstrations, the manufactured gasps about health care costs beget political proposals that beget headlines that beget polls that beget gasps. Hospital people look on and tell one another sadly, "We haven't got our story across to the public."

Whether that is the case or not depends on what it means, and it might mean almost anything. So might the public opinion polls, whose results are determined in large part by the way the questions are asked; an important consideration in interpreting the answers is to know who's asking. At any rate, along with the health care polls that produce gasps there are others with less alarming implications. Thus the Gallup Organization, presumably an unbiased seeker of opinions, recently reported 88 percent of respondents either very satisfied or fairly satisfied with the care they got on their last hospital visit—the same answer that the same question had evoked for the past three years. Asked what were "the main problems facing health care today"—a question that could scarcely be expected to elicit cheers, 65 percent of the respondents mentioned cost first in 1979, compared with 66 percent in 1978 and 49 percent in 1977, an increase, to be sure, but not exactly a gasper, considering what the question was.

Whether we have or haven't got our story across to the public must always be a matter of interpretation, but it is a fact that enough of the story has got across to enough of the people's representatives in the Congress to hold off for three years the legislation that has been feared most. The way things work, the vote could go another way another time no matter who does what, but the experience so far suggests that the important thing may not be getting the story across to the public, whatever that may mean, but getting the right messages to the right people at the right time. This may be harder to do. Almost any information sprayed into the air in hopes that it may land on somebody who is looking or listening can be called telling the hospital story to the public, but getting the message where it counts takes a lot of careful thought, detailed planning, and hard work on the part of everybody from the trustees to the doorman.

This is probably just as true for the individual institution and its community as it is for the entire hospital industry, as it is now unhappily called, and the entire population. Without an information policy established by the board, information goals worked out with the chief executive, and information assistance provided as needed by the departments, the hospital public relations director can still keep busy, and if he knows his job may get a lot of publicity for the hospital and modify the damage on those inevitable occasions when the hospital is in the news and would rather not be. The bad publicity doesn't hurt much, and the good publicity may help some, but in the absence of an overall management public relations plan miscellaneous publicity usually tells people things about the hospital that they already know and doesn't help move the institution any closer to achievement of its goals.

The goals may vary according to the size and nature of the institution and its role in the community, but in every case the principal goals will have to do with patient care, financial security, and future development. Put another way, this means supporting the doctors, finding means of adding revenue and subtracting cost, anticipating the impact of external forces, and making the appropriate countervailing moves. Obviously, these goals and activities are all interrelated, and just as obviously their effective management requires the understanding and accommodation of many different groups, inside and outside the institution, all of which need to be informed in one way or another about the activities that concern them and about the way these activities relate to the institutional mission. "We're involved in the preparation of materials for some 30 separate audiences," the director of community relations at a 400-bed hospital told a visitor recently. "Of course, some of these have about the same content, but you don't tell it the same way to employees and patients, for example. You don't tell the same things to doctors and donors, or even to two different donors, in many cases." That probably isn't what anybody would call telling the hospital story to the public, but it's putting information to work where it will do the most good—for the hospital *and* for the public.

All this isn't to say that press and television aren't as important to hospitals as they are to government, business, or any other establishment in the society. They would all rather be understood than mistrusted, rather appreciated than criticized, and rather seen than ignored. Favorable newspaper stories and broadcasts may contribute something toward the desired dispositions, though never in the way or to the degree that public opinion is instructed by the media to think about wars overseas and politicians underfoot, for the simple but commonly unremarked reason that all we know about wars and politicians is what we read in the papers, but we all know hospitals at first hand as patients or families.

As sources of news, even in periods of international crises, hospitals are not likely to be ignored by the media, but the nature of news is such that the failures are reported on page one and the successes back among the comics, if at all. Managing these occasions so as to achieve the best possible balance of good and bad is a part of the art of hospital public relations—though not the whole of it, or even the greater part, as many suppose. Inevitably, among those who suppose so are some public relations directors themselves who don't know and wouldn't believe that a nice news story or TV report about a child patient or a benefit may make everybody feel good but isn't going to pay any bills or save any lives, and a bad rap in the papers makes everybody furious but doesn't change anything either, and in any case there are other ways of making the messages work.

In a few minutes, any hospital executive can run up an imposing list of people and groups that it would be useful to have better informed than they usually are about the hospital's activities, problems, and goals. The list of insiders would include trustees, doctors, auxiliary members, employees, patients and their families, and visitors. The outside list would begin with donors, prospective donors, and all the relevant public and private parties having something to do with institutional solvency—notably payers and intermediaries, rate review and approval authorities, planning agencies, referral sources, bankers and mortgagees, and others. Appropriate members of legislative bodies would certainly be included, as would other health and social institutions and agencies, employers, unions, civic and social clubs and organizations, consumer groups, and perhaps schools, clergy, and individual community leaders. A sensible information policy would comprehend the kind of information each of these groups should have, and what for, and the function of public relations, in addition to telling the hospital story to the public through the media, would be to devise the best means of getting the messages to the audiences. And as everybody knows, it doesn't do much good to deliver a message once; you have to keep it coming.

In one way or another, most hospitals are doing this, or think they are, though in more cases than not they are probably overlooking some important groups altogether and consider that the job is done for the rest of them when they are sent copies of the annual report, which will tell nearly all these special audiences less than they need to know about their particular interests in the hospital and more than they need to know about everything else. For some of the audiences the most effective means of delivering the message is person-to-person, and in many cases the most effective person to deliver it is the doctor. With patients, families, and donors, and often with legislators, employers, and community leaders, the doctor whose interest can be engaged and put to occasional use can accomplish more in a few minutes' conversation than could be done with a drawerful of letters, brochures, and special reports.

When this possibility has been suggested, the response of some hospital administrators and trustees has been, "Are you kidding? The doctors are the ones who *need* information about the hospital!"

Unquestionably this is true of some doctors in all hospitals, and perhaps of all doctors in some hospitals. But there is reliable research suggesting that physicians are considered by most people in all walks of life to be the most trusted and credible source of information about anything having to do with health, and there are many hospital administrators and trustees who can testify that their doctors have proved to be effective persuaders in dealing with legislators and donors, once they are informed of the hospital's need for support and convinced that a threat to the hospital's independence and solvency is a threat to the doctor's patients and practice. With HSAs breathing heavily on facility and equipment proposals and cost-cap legislation coming on stronger year after year, this proposition isn't as hard to prove as it used to be. Among other things, the voluntary cost containment effort has made a lot of physicians understand that what is bad for hospitals is bad for them—including many who used to think it was just the other way around. Of course, it doesn't follow that the doctor who knows what is good for him is going to be willing to *do* anything about it. But usually one or two can be found who are willing to listen, at least, and then mention some of the hospital's problems to colleagues. With some hints about a few things that need to be known the word may get around, with doctors talking to doctors, that some of the facts ought to be passed along to Very Important Patients. And if somebody keeps feeding the hospital end of the pipeline, without getting pushy about it, this can become an information program. There isn't any way to measure the results, but it might beat headlines.

For one specific purpose, at least, the doctor pipeline is far superior to the headline, or any other method of communication.

That is in engaging the attention, and then the interest, and then the support, of major donors. Almost without exception, hospital fund raisers and development people agree that for fund-raising effectiveness nobody else can match the enthusiastic physician who is willing to talk to his patients about the hospital's need for contributed funds, and ask for help. Of course, not many are, except in those rare cases where the hospital's need for a particular facility or piece of equipment is a perfect fit with the doctor's dream for his own professional interest. This happens often enough to keep fund raisers looking for the combination, and also to keep them searching for the one or two physicians that can often be found who are loyal and conscientious enough to ask for support for the hospital without regard for their own interests. With doctors like that, you've got a running start on telling the hospital story, with or without headlines.

What Are We Doing Here?

The decision by a Federal Trade Commission administrative law judge that the American Medical Association has restricted and frustrated competition in the provision of physicians' services and thus caused substantial injury to the public, while it isn't final and will unquestionably be appealed, may be considered an indication of the increasing disposition of government geniuses and assistant geniuses to ignore the difference between the provision of medical services and the provision of goods and services in commerce and industry. Other signs of the same disposition are in evidence. One is the repeated reference by FTC and HEW functionaries to the supposed lack of competition among hospitals—a misreading of the facts that would be laughable if it weren't so dismaying. Another is the recent proposal within the Health Care Financing Administration to seek revision of the law permitting hospitals to choose their own Medicare intermediaries and to put Medicare contracting on a competitive bid basis, like sewer construction. Still another is the exclusion from government reimbursement formulas of adequate allowances for bad debts and free care and other obligations indigenous to the hospital mission.

These and other indications that the line between serving the public and chasing the dollar is becoming indistinct in the view of the federal establishment are disquieting, but what is even more worrisome is the inclination of many in the traditional hospital culture not only to share these departures from the mode of thought that has prevailed in the past but to encourage them—as in references to the "hospital industry," a term that was formerly used to identify manufacturers and suppliers of hospital equipment and materials but comprehends hospitals themselves in the current usage. The headlong rush to the terminology and practices of marketing, some of which are appropriate and some not, is another symptom of the changing attitude. Another is the concept that "administrator" is a pejorative term that should be superseded by "president" or, in the business vulgate, "CEO," which is not only barbaric but inaccurate, since some administrators are CEOs and some aren't. The mad dash for the new technology is also symptomatic, because the machines that save lives may be outnumbered by those that simply pile up unread printouts. Finally, the total preoccupation with cost suggests that the focus on management of patient care recognizing that money matters have to be considered too is giving way to a focus on money matters recognizing that patient care has to be considered too.

It can be argued that hospitals have more to gain than lose by adopting business attitudes and following business practices, and not just government officials but economists and even some in the professions will argue that the public would be served better if medical and hospital services were advertised and offered for sale competitively, like groceries, so patients and families could shop around and get the best deal for the money. At root, that's what the FTC is driving at in its action against the AMA, and that's the way half the inhabitants of the zoological gardens in Washington would like to see hospitals competing. The other half would like to see hospitals embracing in HSA corridors after signing agreements to close wings. Economists would like to see an HMO on every street corner. Nobody in his right mind wants to oppose the use of efficient business methods in hospitals or insistence on standards imposing reasonable limits on the freedom of physicians to spend out of sight for services of questionable utility, but under today's pressures the effort to curb inefficiencies and extravagances threatens to elevate considerations of cost above considerations of care, a circumstance that would erase the difference between medical services and industry and cause inestimable damage.

Weighing and judging the countervailing values of cost and care are primary responsibilities of physicians in their practices and hospital administrators and trustees in their institutions. Decisions are not difficult to make at the extremes, where luxuries or redundancies are involved, on the one hand, and essentials of care are plainly at stake, on the other. The difficult decisions lie somewhere in between, as the values approach an even balance. "The physician is rightly committed to the best possible care of his or her patient, whether that patient is treated in the elegant supportive environment of our most sophisticated hospital, on a jungle battlefield, or in a good, but less elegant, community hospital," Jacqueline Wexler, president of Hunter College of City University of New York, said in addressing a conference of hospital trustees about the painful moral choices they face at the borderline of cost and care.[1] The low incidence of doctors and patients with spartan attitudes is what makes choices difficult for hospital trustees, Wexler concluded. "Priority decision making within and across societal needs is very tough," she said. "I believe it is probably impossible without rigorous containment of some kind. It is your responsibility as hospital trustees to make that containment rigorous but not rigid."

This is where the difference between medical service and industry has to be put on the scale and weighed, and the difference is measured by the ethical principle that has been a guiding force in medical practice and medical institutions—and not less so because it has been interpreted by the FTC as restrictive on competition or because it is sometimes subordinated to self-interest by physicians and institutions. The principle is simplicity itself: care over cost. As it is set forth in the first section of the AMA's Principles of Medical Ethics, a body of doctrine that is more than 100 years old and deserves more respect than it gets, the principle is also unmistakable: "The principal objective of the medical profession is to render service to humanity with full respect for the dignity of man." It is binding on individual members of the medical profession, and it is equally binding on medical institutions—or else the reason for their existence vanishes and our physicians could as easily render their services in factories or department stores, or city halls. "The difference between industry and a profession is simple," the British philosopher Richard Tawney wrote early in this century. "The essence of the former is that its only criterion is the financial return which it offers to its shareholders. The essence of the latter is that, though men enter it for the sake of livelihood, the measure of their success is the service which they perform, not the gains which they amass."[2]

In a passage that ought to be required reading for hospital administrators and trustees, and officials of HEW and FTC, Tawney continued: "A profession assumes certain responsibilities for the competence of its members or the quality of its wares, and it deliberately prohibits certain kinds of conduct on the ground that, though they may be profitable to the individual, they are calculated to bring into disrepute the organization to which he belongs. The rules themselves may sometimes appear to the layman arbitrary and ill conceived. But their object is clear. It is to impose on the profession itself the obligation of maintaining the quality of the service, and to prevent its common purpose being frustrated through the undue influence of the motive of pecuniary gain." Again, it should be plain that the rules for the medical practitioner must also be the rules for the medical institution. A physician practicing in an institution with an ethic different from his own sooner or later must be either debased, or demoralized, or deceived, and the institution sooner or later must fail the expectations, and ultimately the needs, of its patients.

Why? The reason is that the society, not just in our country in our time but over the world and over the centuries, has had to trust the intention more than the competence of its healers, because it has generally been unable to judge the latter and has come to believe in the former. Our trust is based in the ethic of the healing profession, which was not formulated *de novo* by the founders of the AMA in 1847 but was already well established when St. Luke related the tale of the Good Samaritan. There have been traducers of the trust over the years, and there are some now among practitioners and among institutions, but the ethic still stands, and the society still believes in the intentions of its healers and its healing institutions. Rancorous criticism of hospitals and doctors by government officials, eagerly retailed by press and broadcast media, hasn't made that much difference; the opinion polls still reflect a generous measure of satisfaction with medical services, and any curious legislator or commissioner who wants to question how the society feels about its hospitals should try to close one of them and see what happens.

The threat now is that the profession and its institutions could be pressured into abandoning or blinking at the ethical principle that has been their most distinguishing and ennobling characteristic. The FTC is throwing its weight around and may have overreached in its attack on the AMA, which is focused on advertising for the moment but is obviously intended to diminish the influence of professional associations on professional practices. But the Principles of Medical Ethics do not prohibit advertising; they prohibit solicitation of patients, and the AMA's Judicial Council has explained the difference: "Advertising means making information or intention known to the public, and the physician may furnish this information through the accepted local media," the council said. "Solicitation means the attempt to obtain patients by using statements or claims that (1) contain testimonials, (2) are intended or likely to create inflated or unjustified expectations of favorable results, (3) are self-laudatory and imply that the physician has skills superior to other physicians, or (4) contain incorrect or incomplete facts or representations or implications."[3] It is hard to imagine anything that could destroy public trust more effectively than would be done by allowing or encouraging physicians and hospitals to engage in the practices this principle prohibits, and anybody who doubts that can look at one of those opinion polls that rank public confidence in our institutions. Invariably, medicine is at the top and advertising somewhere near the bottom. The AMA is absolutely right in its determination to fight the FTC decision all the way, and hospitals should make it their fight too. Only physicians and hospital administrators consider that their interests and problems can be viewed separately; everybody else thinks they are identical.

Actually, their interests and problems *are* different at times, as when the physician is convinced that an equipment investment is essential for patient care and the administration and board are convinced that the same investment would be disastrous for institutional solvency. But even these painful occasions can be made less abrasive if the physician remembers that solvency is essential for patient care and the management remembers that patient care is the only reason solvency is important, and they both understand that the decision is not only professional and economic but also moral. The shared ethical principle may not resolve the argument, but it should quiet the shouting. And because trustees have the final responsibility, they need to be aware of an insidious threat that lurks in every decision: the relentless pressure on cost that could erode the cardinal ethic and turn the institution by imperceptible increments until it faced away from its true mission. Given the condition, there may be no way to guard against this hazard, but it might help some if everybody stopped talking about the hospital industry and marketing and the CEO and remembered what it is that we're all doing here. It should be possible for hospitals to borrow what is good about business from business and keep what is best about hospitals for hospitals.

[1]Wexler, J., Remarks presented at the Second National Hospital Trustee Conference, Hunter College Center for Lifelong Learning, New York: December 4, 1978.

[2]Tawney, R.H., The Acquisitive Society, New York: Harcourt, Brace and Company, 1920.

[3]Opinions and Reports of the Judicial Council, prepared and approved by the Judicial Council, Chicago: American Medical Association, 1977.

Of Snake Oil and
Science

April 1978

In a book called *The New Industrial State,* John Kenneth Galbraith, the iconoclastic economist, argues that industry today controls the means for creating the markets for the products its technology makes and is thus in a no-lose position, because it also employs most of the people and pays them the wages they need to buy the products. This control of economic forces could be upset by political upheavals interfering with the flow of resources, such as energy, but to the extent that it is true it may explain the extraordinary ascendancy of marketing executives in our time. Unlike their corporate associates in sales and advertising, whose job is simply to peddle the goods and services their employers produce, the marketing people conduct research to take the temperature of the population; then they take part in planning and promoting the products their thermometers tell them they can profitably sell. As a cynical newsman once observed, the process is one that requires the combined talents of John the Baptist and a Mississippi snake doctor.

The practitioners themselves resent this description, since they like to think of their contribution not as black art but as science. Whatever it is, and it seems likely that it takes something of both art and science, over the past year or two marketing has been invading the hospital field, to the point where it is a rare hospital executive who hasn't attended a seminar or conference where a marketing genius from another industry has been spreading the word about this newly revealed answer to the problems and perplexities of hospitals at a time of crisis, or, at any rate, hypothesized crisis. The effectiveness of these presentations can be measured by the number of hospitals that have introduced the language of marketing into their reports and the number of directors of planning or public relations whose doors and cards bear new titles. This is not bad, because there is always something to be learned from the experience and expertise of others. Like all imports, however, experience and expertise must be introduced by those who understand the language and culture of the receiving country, in order to safeguard against damaging misuse.

Actually, marketing isn't anything new for hospitals, but mostly a new name for what has been a familiar process. Hospitals have been performing the basic tasks of marketing right along—conducting studies to identify the needs of the population, then planning and designing the facilities and services required to meet the needs, and informing the population that the services are there to be used. Thus hospitals, or many if not most of them, have concerned themselves with what is called the marketing mix—product, price, place, and promotion; in the case of hospitals, however, the interplay of these components is less susceptible to being manipulated than it is in other markets.

The components of marketing as it exists in other industries that have not been practiced by hospitals are the planned creation of demand and the aggressive promotion and sale of the goods and services that are produced, and these are the components that offer the greatest hazard of being inappropriately applied to hospitals. In industry, the essential goal of the marketing effort is more—more sales and more profits—and the underlying principle is that more is better. This principle has fueled the growth of the American economy for the past 100 years, at least, so the creation of demand has usually had a legitimate social purpose as well as an obvious corporate purpose. To some extent, the goal of hospital planning for most of those years for most institutions has also been more—more beds and more services. But the time has come now when the goal of planning for hospitals may have to be less, not more, and the principle underlying the planning effort has never been that more is better per se. In the hospital culture, more is better only when quality is assured and only when people need more services. When people need fewer services, as is unquestionably the case now in many areas, less is better. It is ironic that the perceived need in the hospital field for an art built on the principle that more is better should have emerged at precisely the time it is becoming apparent that the reverse may be true.

Now in fairness it must be acknowledged that the burgeoning

literature of marketing generally denies its focus on more and prefers to describe the marketing concept as comprehending the management, not just the creation, of demand. In a recent essay on the subject, in fact, one of the high priests of the art postulated that "to deal effectively with manufacturing, research and development, finance and control, advertising, sales, and market research, the marketing executives should have moved through these departments on the way up. He should understand the problems of these other departments, and they should know that he knows all about their problems." With marketing executives like that, who needs presidents?

The incidence of marketing executives on the presidential model is limited, however; the more familiar figure is the executive who has graduated from an experience in sales, sales management, sales promotion, or advertising, where the watchword is growth and the goal is more. It is no accident, either, that hospitals are grasping for the help offered by marketing consultants at a time when growth is equated with sin. The pressure to hold down or reduce the number of beds has threatened the instinct for institutional survival and sharpened the competitive resolve to make certain by whatever means are at hand that it is somebody else who gets cut off at the knees. The message is clear in a suggestion made by one of the visiting professors from another culture: "Hospitals are looking to the field of marketing," he said, "in hopes of finding a fresh approach to solving the problems of maintaining a productive census level."

That isn't exactly the goal the Congress and the administrators of the planning law had in mind. The creation of demand for hospital services has no legitimate social purpose when it results in the sale of services that are not needed; it is socially useful only in instances where it can uncover a genuine need of which the population has not been aware. This is most likely to occur in places and at economic levels where added hospital census will create more problems than it solves, but in any case the disclosure of needs for medical service is not a simple process of asking questions and counting noses; it is a complex, painstaking task of acquiring and studying data, not to be accomplished by the customary instruments of marketing research except as these are guided by the most knowledgeable and experienced of hospital hands. The demand for health care is influenced by all the factors the economists have recognized:

availability, access, cost, insurance, physicians' decisions, internal and external controls of all kinds. But the basic determinant of use is epidemiology—how many people get sick or hurt and need care—and epidemiology is not responsive to the ministrations of marketing. So what the new marketing maneuvers may come down to in more cases than not is finding ways of persuading Physician A to favor Hospital X over Hospital Y, a process that may reward one institution at the expense of another and can also be damaging to the health economy as a whole when the lure includes some consideration of added facilities, equipment, or personnel.

This is not what the planning law contemplated, either, and it is not what Congress and the Federal Trade Commission are looking for when they deplore what they see as lack of competition among hospitals. The fact is that hospitals are about as competitive as you can get, short of assassination, and it is the competition itself, and not the absence of it, that is responsible for many of the excesses now causing wringing of hands in the offices and corridors of government. The competition is responsible for excellence as well as excess and is thus to be discouraged only at some risk, but those who share the simplistic view that advertising by hospitals and doctors will stimulate competition and bring costs down are precisely and disastrously wrong. The patient choosing a physician doesn't shop around for a bargain, as he might do when choosing a carpenter or cobbler, and the physician choosing a hospital doesn't care about price, because he doesn't pay. It can be argued that it would be better if this were not so, but the argument doesn't alter the circumstance that the demand for care, unlike the demand for cars, is related only distantly to cost. There is no price tag on epidemiology, and competition among providers can be an added cost.

So can advertising. We have seen now what happened in California when the FTC, like a bull in a blood bank, started breaking up the furniture with its charges about AMA suppression of advertising by doctors. The ones who started advertising were the borderline surgeons aiming at volume in elective procedures. Within a few weeks, promoters came out of the woodwork to advertise surgical centers or clearinghouses, contracting with the surgeons to wield their questionable skills and scalpels. It seems likely that the same thing would happen to hospitals if all the constraints arising from the nature of the hospital mission were to be removed. The grabbers and the trimmers would burgeon, the reputable core would suffer losses of patronage and esteem, and the patients of the grabbers and trimmers would just suffer. The reason this would happen is clear to everybody except those who are pushing for doctors and hospitals to compete by cutting prices, the way gas stations and supermarkets do: Advertising doesn't change the epidemiology, and those who get sick or hurt have no sensible way to judge the value of medical services, let alone strike a balance of value and price, as they commonly do in the case of dresses and deodorants. So they have to trust the intentions as well as the competence of their physicians and institutions, and this trust imposes on physicians and hospitals the obligation that is the bedrock of the professional ethic. The obligation and the ethic that emerges from it measure the difference between hospitals and industry, and nowhere more obtrusively than in marketing.

This is not to say that there should be no marketing or advertising by hospitals. The research and planning functions of marketing are essential elements of hospital operations, and the information and advertising functions of marketing are essential elements of sound public policy for hospitals. In all these functions, it makes good sense for hospitals to seek advice and assistance from marketing talent in other industries, exercising the providence suggested by a visiting professor: "The basic requirements for effective marketing within the health organization are an attitude of responsiveness toward the needs and perceptions of all its constituencies, and specific competence in carrying out marketing tasks. . . . Marketing in the health field has unique properties which challenge conventional marketing principles and require intelligent adaptations rather than automatic implementation."[1]

In the past, the requisite talents have usually been available from hospital trustees recruited with some awareness of their expertise, and this is still the case in many institutions. Where it isn't, there is no reason hospitals shouldn't seek out and pay for marketing services as they do for financial, architectural, engineering, or any other technical or professional advice. But whether the help is volunteered or paid for, the important thing is that it should be applied within the limitations established by the ethic that marks the difference between hospitals and other industry. The "fresh approach to solving the problems of maintaining a productive census level" is marketing language that could suggest either legitimate hospital planning or the slick come-on of a Mississippi snake doctor. The executive in the hospital environment would always know the difference. The professor from another country might not.

[1]MacStravic, R.E., Marketing Health Care, Germantown, MD: Aspen Systems Corp., 1977.

Forty Years of
Trial and Error

December 1978

Some 40 years ago, give or take, I spent a large part of my time for several years in work that could be called health education of the public—an exercise that is finally emerging from the dusty cubby-holes of public health departments and the spare-time attention of physical education teachers, and commanding the serious interest of health professionals, educators, government officials, and business executives, all of whom in increasing numbers are coming to realize that health care costs can never be controlled by beating down providers, without some corresponding effort to persuade consumers to shape up and stay well. There are many skeptics still in the professions, in government, and in industry, but there is also a real push now to examine what needs to be done to inform and motivate the population to accept greater responsibility for its own health, and know what to do about it. It is a basic assumption that these are desirable goals, though there is some disagreement about the extent to which consideration should be given, in all prudence, to the use of hospital resources for purposes whose ultimate result would appear to be to empty the beds the hospital has to keep full in order to earn the revenue it has to have to do all the other things it is expected to do. Under the circumstances, it is remarkable that so many hospitals have been willing to join the effort, and it is possible that a brief look at some of our experiences in the Dark Ages may help these hospitals now to avoid the more egregious of our mistakes.

In my experience as a health educator, I had three different assignments. One was as editor of a community hospital publication that was basically an instrument of fund raising but one of whose purposes, by specific direction of the board of trustees, was to inform readers on matters of health and medicine. Another task of those years was as associate editor of *Hygeia,* a magazine published by the American Medical Association, later known as *Today's Health*, and last seen disappearing from the AMA into another, similar enterprise. In a third assignment of that depression-ridden era, I was a ghostwriter, or more accurately a ghostwriter's ghostwriter, in a stable employed by a celebrated physician-politician who was public health commissioner of a large city and whose literary cartel included a daily syndicated health column that appeared in several hundred newspapers around the country, a monthly article in a national woman's magazine with a circulation in millions, and an unending flow of books, pamphlets, manuals, and tracts on maternal and infant welfare and child care—then as now a guaranteed method of grabbing an audience.

The health education vehicle in the first instance, the community hospital publication, was chiefly interviews with members of the hospital's medical staff, the idea being that the readers would thereby gain some useful knowledge about health and medicine and at the same time be subtly reminded that the hospital represented a vast reservoir of medical knowledge and skill, always on tap in the community. This proposition seemed logical enough on the face of it but unfortunately neglected to consider that the interviews inevitably consisted for the most part of things the doctors thought the people ought to know, and there was never any evidence that these were the things the people wanted to know, a disjunction that proved difficult to avoid and was discouraging, not to say fatal, to effective communication. Unhappily, this mismating of purpose and method is still apparent in a substantial fraction of the information that is sprayed into the air in the name of health education of the public.

The same disjunction existed at *Hygeia*, though to a lesser degree because the chief editor was smart enough to understand that there were more people who wanted to know what to do about athlete's foot than there were people who wanted to know about the latest research in schistosomiasis. But the standard fare at *Hygeia* was still "New Hope for Millions of Sufferers," interlarded with copy prepared by the AMA's health education staff dealing with how to take care of everything from the toes to the scalp. The articles were loaded with practical information, but the problem was that whenever there was anything seriously wrong with the part under consideration, policy required that in order to avoid upsetting physicians in private practice the article had to back off and not tell the reader much of anything except that he should hustle down and consult his own physician. It wasn't bad advice, but it wasn't what readers were looking for, either. The only exception to the rule was articles about nutrition, which were considered outside the physician's jurisdiction then, as they are for the most part still, so we could tell readers anything there was to know about what and when and how to eat in order to be healthy. The flaw in the formula was that in those days, before yogurt and granola and wheat germ and Adele Davis were invented, nobody really wanted to read about nutrition.

By far the most effective of the health educators I was involved with was the physician-politician, who understood exactly what mothers wanted to know about taking care of their babies and told them in great detail, unabashed by the dictum against giving away the kind of advice that was considered to be within the domain of the physician in private practice. In fact, the columns and articles we produced were frequently cited by the local medical society as violating its principles of ethics, in the quaint professional meaning of the term, but the commissioner couldn't have cared less. The first time the question was raised, he resigned from the society. This maneuver was conducted in a fashion to make it appear that the society was somehow bent on preventing a public benefactor from bringing enlightenment to the masses—a posture that medical societies have not yet completely mastered the art of avoiding.

All the mistaken notions we had about health education a generation ago are still around, to be sure, but along with so much wasted effort there are now many new programs combining modern information techniques with some soundly based knowledge, limited but growing, about what it takes to motivate people to change their behavior. For example, we have learned by trial and error that information alone doesn't accomplish much of anything unless it is accompanied by some galvanizing force that induces action, and we have learned also that unless the flow of information and motivating incentive can be sustained, any change in behavior that may result is likely to be short-lived. It was reported that Mrs. Gerald Ford's mastectomy sent thousands of women to doctors' offices, clinics, and hospitals all over the country for breast examinations, but the number seeking care dropped right back down again as soon as Mrs. Ford was out of the news. It can be argued that the one-time surge may have accomplished something worthwhile for the health of American women, but it is also unarguable that something more would be accomplished if we could find an equivalent to Mrs. Ford for every month of the year.

It isn't impossible. The Stanford Heart Study has produced a hierarchy of changed eating, drinking, smoking, and exercising behaviors—a little change in the community where messages in the mass media were used and repeated, a lot more change where the messages were reinforced by face-to-face consultations. The Health Hazard Appraisal invented by Drs. Lewis Robbins and Jack Hall of Indianapolis, a method now used regularly by several hundred practicing physicians throughout the country, brings to bear an effective personalized motivator in the physician's promise to add years to the patient's life span if he agrees to abide by rules of living based on mortality and morbidity statistics, such as cancer and heart disease rates for smokers and nonsmokers. The statistics are studied by patient and physician together and applied to the patient's own life situation. Another kind of motivation has been reported by Dr. Keith W. Sehnert, who taught his patients in a Virginia suburb of Washington to do a lot of things for themselves and wrote a book about it,[1] and by Dr. Ross Egger, a general practitioner in a small town in Indiana who has 4,000 patients but sees only 22 of them a day in his office because he has spent a lot of time over the years teaching them how to take care of themselves unless they're in real trouble, and how to tell when they are, in which case they're more likely to call up than to come in. About 60 patients call up on an average day, Dr. Egger reported, and his nurse usually handles 40 of them by herself. "I talk to about 20 of them," he said. "I don't mind it at all because it makes my job easier. The patient is participating in his care to the same degree that I am. It's a matter of us deciding together what will help him."[2] Some patients don't like it that way, he has acknowledged, and usually they manage to find another doctor—one who doesn't like it that way either. A lot of doctors think teaching patients to take care of themselves is like teaching the passengers to fly the airplane.

It would seem that the strongest imaginable motivator and reinforcer of good health behavior should be at work in the patient who has something seriously the matter with him and knows it. We all want to stick around. But the elusive quality of motivation is apparent in the fact that even these patients don't always take care of themselves, as in the case of smokers with chronic obstructive pulmonary disease and hypertensives who don't renew their prescriptions. The best explanation of this irrational behavior is probably the one offered by Dr. Ernst Wynder, president of the American Health Foundation, who has called it the illusion of immortality. "They simply don't believe it can happen to them," he said. For this and other reasons, behavioral scientists are beginning to doubt the efficacy of fear as an incentive to healthier living. Campaigns emphasizing early symptoms of cancer or heart disease may scare as many patients away from doctors as they send to see doctors, it is suggested, and at least one carefully conducted opinion poll has demonstrated that the public knowledge of health hazards is way ahead of the public observance of good health habits.[3]

These and other barriers to effective health education, such as television entertainment glorifying violence and excess and television advertising glamorizing useless or harmful products, are discouraging but not insuperable obstacles to those who are initiating the new information and motivation programs in industry and the professions. Industry abounds with programs that screen employed groups to identify problems and provide appropriate corrective, supportive, and educational services; Blue Cross Plans and insurance companies are providing educational materials for subscribers and policyholders; hospitals are extending educational activities from the bedside to outpatient departments and in some cases to whole communities; legislative proposals are appearing that would add education and incentive components, as well as cost containment strictures, to government programs. The new fitness mania is exemplified in the jogging phenomenon, which is now reaching millions and may yet prove to be the means by which good health is made fashionable—a result that would probably make all the other incentives redundant.

For some years now, many leaders of hospital thought have been saying that the proper function of the hospital in society is to serve as the central focus for all health care activities in the community it serves, rather than simply as the repository or recourse for the acutely ill and injured. The fact that most hospitals have remained more of the latter than the former needn't be considered an indication of failure or dereliction; care of the sick and injured is a necessary and noble contribution to the well-being of the society. But for those institutions that aspire to be a true center or focus of health care activity, there can be no blinking the responsibility for using their considerable resources of knowledge and talent to enlighten their constituencies and communities on matters related to health. In fact, the view that *all* hospitals share this responsibility was emphasized at the 1978 convention of the American Hospital Association by such AHA luminaries as Gail Warden and H. Robert Cathcart. Thus it seems likely that many more hospitals will be doing in coming months what some have already started to do and a few have been doing right along—distributing publications and films for public audiences, offering facilities and talent for use by community groups, assisting other agencies and organizations in planning and conducting education programs, consulting with employers, educators, and others with an interest in improving the health status of the population, taking pains to set an example as an employer by offering such service for their employees and staff. Hospitals that really mean it can be expected to carefully monitor the foods served to the public in cafeterias and snack bars, and to discontinue the sale of cigarettes and restrict smoking to sharply defined and limited areas—at whatever pain of disaffection by visitors.

None of these things are easy to do, and they are especially difficult to keep on doing in the absence of any solid evidence that they are accomplishing something worthwhile. Dr. Ernst Wynder likes to tell employers that the entire cost of the screening and preventive education service offered by the American Health Foundation for a group of 1,500 employees, say, will be saved if it results in avoiding a single coronary bypass operation—an impressive statistic unless the employer stops to consider that he'll never know whether a coronary bypass was avoided or not. Evaluating health education outcomes is an arcane art, as one of its leading practitioners, Dr. Lawrence W. Green of the Johns Hopkins School of Hygiene and Public Health, has explained. "We are sometimes guilty of claiming too much for health education, as we do when we give the impression that educational effects are usually permanent," he said in a paper describing what is known about the art. "In fact, we know a great deal about learning curves and memory curves, and the process of forgetting and backsliding. We know that reinforcement is as important to education as booster shots are to sustained immunization."[4] Until more specific data can be accumulated in controlled studies now being conducted in several centers, "assumptions based on theory and experience must suffice," Dr. Green concluded.

Meanwhile, changes in behavior can be observed over time in most hospital programs and communities, and in large groups over long periods outcomes can be evaluated in terms of morbidity, hospital days used, readmission rates, and other indicators. And if every one of those millions of men and women who are causing traffic jams as they jog through the nation's streets and parks would knock off a few blocks and spend the time they save writing or calling their TV stations to protest the ads for soft drinks, candy bars, sugar-coated this and deep-fried that, they might accomplish more to improve the nation's health than all the health education programs have done—over these 40 years of trial and, mostly, error.

[1]Sehnert, K., with Eisenberg, H., How To Be Your Own Doctor Sometimes, New York: Grosset & Dunlap, 1975.

[2]Egger, R.L., I Make My Patients Be Their Own Doctors, Medical Economics 55:83, June 12, 1978.

[3]Louis Harris Report for Mount Sinai Hospital Medical Center, Chicago, January 1977.

[4]Green, L.W., Evaluation and Measurement: Some Dilemmas for Health Education. Presented in part at the Midwest Conference on Health Education sponsored by the University of Illinois School of Public Health, Chicago: June 2, 1976

Keeping Them Well Is Good Business Too

October 1979

Take a walk through almost any city park early on a sunny morning and you're sure to see squads of men and women jogging the perimeter walks and paths and, in the open spaces, here and there a solitary figure, or perhaps a small group, frozen in odd posture—leaning slightly forward, knees bent, arms extended, and, if you watch closely, perhaps slowly raising an arm or leg or otherwise showing that is is not, as you may have thought at first, immobile. Strangely, as it turns out, the joggers and the slow-motion exercisers may be pursuing similar goals. Most joggers call theirs fitness and measure it in pulse and respiration rates and diastolic pressure, and the more dedicated runners refer to the onset of a kind of clarity of mind and spirit unlike anything experienced at shorter distances and lesser speeds. This rapture of the runners may be akin to the Supreme Ultimate, or Way, sought by the moving statues, who are performing T'ai-Chi, a Chinese practice having its roots in the Taoist belief that man and the universe conform to the same rhythms. The T'ai-Chi movements, following a coordinated rhythmic pattern and performed in sequence, are thought to produce the inner void that permits man to return to nature's origin, in harmony with the universe.

"The basic difference between the Chinese and the Western systems of exercises is that the Chinese exercises are linked with philosophy," said K.K. Jain, M.D., a neurosurgeon who was born in India, educated in the United States, and practices in Canada. "The Western system is purely physical. It is easy to evaluate these exercises by the standard laboratory methods to determine their effect on the body. It is a little more difficult to determine the effect of the Chinese system of exercises, for example the T'ai-Chi, since there have been no scientific studies to measure body functions of a person doing T'ai-Chi exercises."[1] But T'ai-Chi is similar to Yoga, Dr. Jain said, and the All-India Institute of Medical Science has made extensive studies of yogis doing their exercises. "It has been shown that a yogi can control his pulse and breathing and slow down his metabolic rate to a point where he could survive without oxygen for a much longer period than is commonly considered compatible with life. Electroencephalograms done during these exercises indicate slowing of brain activity and a state of ideal mental relaxation. Using this as an example, one can postulate that the Chinese system of exercise has a somewhat similar purpose in regulating the body. That the performers feel better after these exercises is beyond doubt. A Chinese practicing T'ai-Chi may feel well and be able to maintain mental tranquility in spite of the disturbing external environment."

Reports like this may be expected to evoke mixed response in our time, when most of us would question the usefulness, if not the sanity, of trying to survive without oxygen for a much longer period than is commonly considered compatible with life, and slowing one's brain activity is not a widely coveted talent, except among insomniacs. At the same time, we need all the help we can get in maintaining mental tranquility in spite of the disturbing environment, and the runners should be pleased to know that the elevated state of mind they experience with extreme exertion may actually be oneness with the universe. Short of these exalted goals, there is still something to be said for simple fitness, and for doing whatever can be done now to keep at arm's length the ailments that are going to do us all in eventually, no matter what.

There's a lot to be done. The number of persons taking some kind of regular exercise has been increasing, as the evidence of the parks suggests, but it is still estimated at only a third of the population, and the chances are good that a substantial fraction of those who report "regular exercise" are counting a game of catch with Junior and a walk around the block with the dog. And even if the entire population were put on a strenuous regimen of push-ups, or worse, it would take a while for fitness to get a foothold. As it turns out, we are not in all that great shape. According to an insurance company survey, something more than 60 percent of U.S. adults are overweight, and while most of them say they have been on a diet at one time or another, only one in five was dieting at the time of the survey, and in the absence of a more precise definition than that, it can probably be assumed that dieting for some consists of refusing second helpings of dessert.

Fifty-seven million Americans smoke; 70 percent of them know they may be risking their health, but they smoke anyway. While the number of smokers among adult males has been reduced over the past decade, the number of teenagers who smoke has been increasing, so the total has stayed about the same. Sixteen percent of families report having at least one member who drinks too much; the number having a lush they don't want to talk about is not known, but it has been estimated that fewer than one out of every five of those with a drinking problem have asked for help. Overweight, smoking, and drinking have all been associated with high blood pressure, and this is important because high blood pressure "is at all ages powerfully related to risk of premature major catastrophes—sudden death, heart attack, congestive heart failure, stroke, and kidney failure," according to Jeremiah Stamler, M.D., professor and chairman of the department of community health and preventive medicine at Northwestern University Medical School.[2] Another hypertension specialist, Frank A. Finnerty Jr., of the Washington, DC, Hypertension Center, estimated that the problems resulting from hypertension cause 150 million disability days and 26 million hospitalization days every year, cost business and industry 52 million man days of productivity, and account for the largest number of disability claims under Social Security, which is also currently spending $6 million a week for dialysis for end-stage renal disease, a common consequence of hypertension.[3]

Finnerty is concerned that patients with hypertension but without symptoms are hard to find and hard to treat because they may feel fine and stop taking pills, and for the same reasons doctors are more interested in patients who hurt, and they often fail to notice that a large number of hypertension patients don't return for checkups. Stamler is concerned about these things too, but under the best of circumstances, he believes, "no one can be satisfied with a decades-long perspective of treating millions of hypertensives with drugs. That cannot be the final answer." Progress depends in part on research in the causes of essential hypertension, Stamler said, "but data are extant now on risk factors, including controllable risk factors, for hypertension itself—for example, obesity, high salt intake, rapid heart rate, as well as levels of blood pressure in the high-normal range. And evidence is also available indicating that moderate weight loss is associated with significant lowering of blood pressure and prevention of progressive rise over years for persons with high-normal diastolic pressures as well as for those with frank elevations. . . . The data also suggest that improvement in cardiopulmonary fitness achieved by regular frequent moderate rhythmic exercise, with consequent slowing of casual heart rate, contributes to prevention of evolution to frank hypertension for persons with high-normal diastolic pressures. These facts point to the possibility of implementing approaches now that may accomplish the primary prevention of hypertension by safe nutritional-hygienic means—especially for hypertension-prone people, but also for the population at large, through general improvement in the norms of life style."

Given that a large segment of the population would benefit from losing weight, eating sensibly, smoking and drinking less, and exercising more, what can be done about it? The health care literature is loaded with reports of studies showing that people can be informed and motivated to change their behavior along the lines suggested by Stamler and others, but the experience of physicians and health educators also suggests that if the educational programs are not sustained and the motivating influences not periodically reinforced, behavior is likely to revert to former patterns. An executive associated with one of the most popular, and profitable, weight control systems reported, for example, that the recidivism rate among its clientele was generally in excess of 90 percent; everybody who has ever smoked knows that it is easy to quit but hard to stay quit; drinkers fall off the wagon almost as often as they climb back on, and the jogger traffic in the parks vanishes in cold or rainy weather, suggesting that the motivation is something less than compelling—or perhaps that for most of its practitioners jogging lacks the link to philosophy that dignifies T'ai-Chi.

What, then? One reason people who know better don't take care of themselves, or start to but don't keep it up, is that they don't have enough trust in their sources of information. In the insurance company survey referred to here, only a third of the respondents felt that public service messages and publications of the American Heart Association, American Cancer Society, and like organizations were useful and reliable sources of information about health, and even fewer believed what they read about health in newspapers and magazines and saw on television. Government publications, advertising, and insurance company booklets were far down the list of credible sources, and employers, unions, friends, and neighbors were at the very end.[4] In contrast, 70 percent of those queried said their own doctors would be considered useful and reliable sources, although less than half of them said they were actually getting much information about health from their doctors. Commenting on this finding, the research organization said: "Many surveys have demonstrated the high regard most people have for their own doctors and the high public trust in the medical opinions and expertise of their doctors. This prevailing attitude could be applied, to a far greater extent than has been done in the past, to change the diet habits and life styles of most Americans. The data demonstrate the enormous importance of the doctor in providing not just medication and treatment but advice and counseling to prevent disease."

The problem is that it isn't easy to provide advice and counseling for people who aren't there. Most doctors are conscientious about instructing the patients who come to them for treatment, as long as they are being treated, but people who think they are well, as most of us do most of the time, stay away from doctors, who aren't very interested in well people anyway. With a few notable exceptions, for the most part among pediatricians and obstetricians, physicians spring to life in the presence of pathology and die of boredom when anybody mentions prevention, a subject associated with public hygiene, sanitation, water supply, immunization and other concerns now of those classmates who had a hard time memorizing the names of the long muscles back in medical school. This results not so much from disinterest in health as from intensified interest in illness as medical science keeps on finding new causes for our ailments and developing new technologies for coping with them. With people believing only doctors who aren't interested, or haven't time, to provide the information and encouragement they need to get healthier and stay that way, the opportunity for hospitals to broaden their usefulness and serve the whole population, and not just the ailing, should be obvious. Most of the rest of us see the hospital as representing, if not belonging to, the doctors, and we are ready to give it the same status and credibility we give them as benefactors of society—a privilege some hospital administrators and trustees seem determined to repudiate by emphasizing their separateness instead of their identity with physicians. Others see their mission as limited to acute care of the ill and injured and aren't any more interested in well people than doctors are; a few consider that hospitals engaging in preventive or health education activities, are simply cutting down the market for their services or emptying the beds they ought to be keeping full.

An increasing number of hospitals, however, have taken the view that the health of the population is a hospital responsibility. In this perspective, motivating people to take better care of themselves, and teaching them how, is as much a part of the hospital mission as repairing the damage when they don't. These hospitals encourage their doctors, nurses, technicians, and others to make information a component of patient care. Using their medical and nursing staffs as resource, they take instruction about good health habits to the whole community in meetings, good health publications and exhibits, and in special events and programs planned with schools, public health departments, and social welfare agencies. Realizing that hospital management isn't news but hospital medicine often is, they seek and make opportunities for the media to report what their doctors and nurses are doing to make their communities healthier and keep them that way. The hospital that is doing all these things may be doing itself out of a few coronary bypass operations a few years from now, but meanwhile it will have made its good works known to many physicians and patients and others who will have chosen it when hospital services are required. This is as good an exercise for hospitals as T'ai-Chi is for men and women, and like T'ai-Chi it is linked to a philosophy: Cast thy bread upon the waters, for it will return after many days.

[1]Jain, K., Health Care in New China and What We Can Learn From It, Emmaus, PA: Rodale Press, Inc., 1973.

[2]Stamler, J., Epidemiology and Treatment of Hypertension, in Carlson, R., ed., Future Directions in Health Care: A New Public Policy, Cambridge, MA: Ballinger Publishing Company, 1978.

[3]Finnerty, F., Use of Paramedical Personnel in Treating Hypertension, in Carlson, R., ed., Future Directions in Health Care: A New Public Policy, Cambridge, MA: Ballinger Publishing Company, 1978.

[4]Health Maintenance, A Nationwide Survey of the Barriers Toward Better Health and Ways of Overcoming Them. Conducted by Louis Harris and Associates, Inc., for Pacific Mutual Life Insurance Company, November 1978.

GOVERNANCE AND MANAGEMENT

What Makes Workers Work?

May 1978

At a time when there is a psychiatrist at every newsstand, a philosopher driving every cab, and an author on every TV program telling you how to rearrange your attitude and your life for greater productivity, happiness, and cash flow, it isn't surprising that the lectures, courses, and institutes for executives and managers are moving off the familiar precincts of planning, organizing, allocating, and controlling, and onto the headier ground of human relations, where anything goes. The journals of management in recent years have been reading more and more like *Psychology Today* or Ann Landers, and the encounter groups whose members are encouraged to bare their inmost secrets to strangers, and to probe for theirs, are moving east from Mill Valley. They haven't got to Wall Street yet, but they're on the way. Young people, especially, judging from their conversation, spend a measurable fraction of their time worrying about their own identities, or, as they say, trying to find out who they are. It's a problem we older types never had to face. There was always somebody around to tell us, and if we didn't like it we knew what we could do.

It isn't easy now to figure out just how, or when, the balance of initiative got shifted, but however it happened it is clear today that in more cases than not it is the boss, and not the employee, who knows what he can do if he doesn't like it. He can take it and shut up, that's what, because if he doesn't he's going to find himself in a meeting with the company psychologist, or the organizational development consultant, or somebody else whose clubby manner is all it takes to get the message across: Managerial attitudes and values are changing, and we are creating an organizational climate characterized by openness and collaboration. Control is out, and participation is in. A worker whose job doesn't meet his need for social acceptance and ego satisfaction, as well as money, isn't likely to be productive, and a manager who doesn't understand these values is out of step with the way things are going.

Well, there isn't much question that this is the way things have been going for the past 20 years, at least. The library shelves are stacked with books and journals explaining the new management theories and reporting where and how and with what success they have been put into practice, and the old-fashioned manager or supervisor who cosseted his favorites and threatened laggards and dissenters is as out-of-date as the rolltop desk. When he retires or has a stroke—the eventuality that may be the more likely—his replacement is going to be young enough to have grown up with parents who avoided disciplining their children for fear of traumatizing their little egos, and teachers who believed the kids were experiencing social adjustment to their peers when they belted each other with the sandbox. The young business school graduates who are climbing the managerial ladders today know all about organizational climate and motivational psychology, or what makes people work. They know, for example, that "the force on a person to perform an act is a monotonically increasing function of the algebraic sum of the valences of all outcomes and the strength of his expectancies that the act will be followed by the attainment of these outcomes," which is the way a distinguished professor of psychology who is also a consultant to industry talks when he wants to say that people will do whatever looks good to turn out the way they want it to.

This principle has never been exactly a secret, but its applicability in an organized way in the working environment may be considered relatively new, possibly beginning in the 1920s in the celebrated experiments with the work force at the Hawthorne Works of the Western Electric Company at Cicero, IL, where the motivating influences of *esprit* or morale consistently outperformed all other incentives to productivity, including money. A German psychologist who came to this country in the 1930s, Kurt Lewin, experimented further with the concept that came to be known as group dynamics, and Lewin's associates, students, followers, and imitators have been spreading the word and elaborating the principles ever since. Some of the variations are now soundly established in common management practice, where the bull-in-a-china-shop tactics of executives who like to think of themselves as hard-nosed have given way steadily to routine assessment of the human as well as the fiscal consequences before decisions are made. But the antics of some of Lewin's ideological descendants have given humanism a bad name at times, as when consultants confuse participation with authority and consider that observance of the psychological principle requires a vote by all hands in advance of every change, or when the psychologist or "facilitator" knows all the theories but lacks the sensitivity to understand that first names and shirtsleeves may be an impediment to achievement of the desirable organizational climate in a business culture accustomed to vests and formalities. Under these circumstances, the unresponsiveness a consultant may read as fear or repression may be simply embarrassment caused by his own behavior.

Psychologic consultants and modern executives who have sense enough to know that you can't lay on the kind of quick-acting technique that will transform managers who are naturally shy into outgoing personality types understand also that this wouldn't do any good anyway. What is needed is not simply a change in management behavior or administrative style, but rather an extension or enlargement of the attitude or focus of management to comprehend goals that generally have been considered irrelevant in the past but are seen increasingly as central to the purposes of most organizations. Heightened job satisfaction is an end in itself, because the organization today is considered to owe a duty to its people as well as to its owners and customers. In addition, and what is more important to managers of the old school for whom people are just one of the components to be manipulated, like money and machines, it is becoming clearer all the time that workers who like what they're doing get more done. Job satisfaction is cost-effective.

As we have seen, you can't just go out and buy a new work environment or hire consultants to install one, like a computer system. Actually, the whole subject of work as an element in the quality of life, and of health, is a lot more complicated than even many of the experts have understood. "However deeply we may have cared in the past, we never really understood the importance, the meaning, and the reach of work," Elliot L. Richardson wrote in 1972 when he was Secretary of Health, Education, and Welfare. As Secretary he had appointed a task force to examine the impact of work on the nation's health, education, and welfare problems, and the task force report—like most government studies of the kind widely unread and ignored—remains a comprehensive review of knowledge on the subject. "This report warns us of the great disservice done to the American people when we ignore the enormous contributions of work to health and education and concentrate instead on medical care and schooling," Richardson continued in his foreword. "We shall make very large mistakes if we fail to pay continuing and close heed to our basic institutions—work, family, and community. This report draws our attention back to matters from which we have been perilously estranged."[1]

In its year-long study, the task force, which was headed by a social anthropologist, found that significant numbers of American workers are dissatisfied with the quality of their working lives. "This is not so much because work itself has greatly changed," the report said. "Indeed, one of the main problems is that work has not changed fast enough to keep up with the rapid and wide-scale changes in worker attitudes, aspirations, and values. Many workers at all occupational levels feel locked in, their mobility blocked, the opportunity to grow lacking in their jobs, challenge missing from their tasks. Young workers appear to be as committed to the institution of work as their elders have been, but many are rebelling against the anachronistic authoritarianism of the workplace." Moreover, the task force found a growing body of research indicating that as these problems multiply there may be a consequent decline in physical and mental health, family stability, community participation, and "balanced socio-political attitudes"—as well as absenteeism, turnover, strikes, sabotage, poor quality products, and "reluctance by workers to commit themselves to their tasks."

Another observer reached a similar conclusion about work. "Voluntary absenteeism has become a great worry to both public and private bureaucracies," Richard Sennett, New York University professor of sociology, said in a recent essay. "Workers often pretend to be sick so they can take paid sick leave. White-collar employees simply disappear for the day or lie about things they need to do outside the office. As the scale of the problem has grown, the perception of it has changed. Personnel experts no longer regard it as simple delinquency but rather as a tactic of resistance—to pressure at the office, to tedium on the assembly line. The corollary, however unpalatable to the managers, has also become unavoidable to them: There must be something wrong at work if so many people are trying to get away from it. The rising volume of these practices has made it untenable to view such workers simply as isolated misfits."[2]

Some of the experts are convinced that it doesn't have to be that way, and that work can be used to alleviate the problems it may be causing and become instead, in the words of the HEW report, "a singularly powerful source of psychological and physical rewards." Several dozen well-documented experiments show that productivity increases and social problems decrease when workers participate in the work decisions affecting their lives, the report said, and when their responsibility for their work is buttressed by participation in profits. What is required to bring about the results is a lot more than the kind of cosmetic change that is often passed off as "job enrichment," the task force concluded. It is the substantive redesign of work and responsibility, and it isn't easy to do. The study group examined and reported what had been done, and with what results, in some three dozen specific cases in U.S. and European industries, ranging from the complete redesign of a food manufacturing plant to the comparatively simple reorganization of a janitorial service into "cleaning teams" that planned and assigned their own jobs and got one-third more work done with a few more than half as many people.

How? In each case, with variations depending on the nature of the enterprise and the type of work, the task force found workers participating in decisions having to do with their own production methods, the internal distribution of tasks, recruitment, internal leadership, additional tasks to take on, and assignments of working time. "Not all the work groups make all these decisions," the report said, "but this is the range within which the workers are participating in the management of the business. Participative management does *not* mean participation through representatives; that kind of participation may foster alienation through the inevitable gap between expected and actual responsiveness of the representatives. Nor does this kind of participation mean placing workers or union representatives on the board of directors. . . . It means that workers are enabled to control the aspects of work intimately affecting their lives. It permits the worker to achieve and maintain a sense of personal worth and importance, to grow, to motivate himself, and to receive recognition and approval for what he does."

Lest anybody should get the wrong idea, this section of the report ends with a reminder that management still runs the enterprise, and that "the concept of work design also needs to be applied to management, where participation also can usefully be increased. The work of managers needs to be redesigned not only because it is unlikely for authoritarian managers to support the humanization of work for lower-level workers, but also for their own physical and mental health. . . . Some steps are already being taken to provide greater job satisfaction for managers, including the decentralization of authority to middle and lower managers, and the formation of teams of managers to solve specific, non-recurrent problems." The lofty aim of these maneuvers was described by Professor Sennett: "Many corporations are attempting to put into practice a new ideology of work," he said, "an ideology of communication, cooperation, and personal growth for the employees. Work comes close to being a form of psychotherapy, and bosses become like analysts."

Bosses playing analyst may be considered a doubtful improvement over bosses playing autocrat, but there isn't any question that the move away from authoritarian management is gaining headway in industry. However, there may be some who would question whether it is equally appropriate for hospitals, where management resides in an environment that must also accommodate the practices of medicine and nursing, whose rigid hierarchies of authority are seen as needed safeguards for standards of patient care—the same argument that is often considered conclusive against the acceptance of unions in hospitals. The countervailing arguments are simply that participation doesn't mean giving away the store and that patient care is improved, not threatened, when workers feel better about their work. It can also be argued persuasively that work redesign may be the best of all ways to retard the rise of unionism in hospitals, where that is regarded as desirable. "To keep non-union workers relatively satisfied," a recent article on the subject said, "companies are using a variety of techniques, including periodic surveys of employee attitudes, training programs to upgrade skills, complaint-airing sessions, worker participation in decision making, and formal systems of step-by-step hearing modeled on union grievance procedures."[3]

Sennett, for one, isn't sure any of this is going to work for very long. "The very nature of this new ideology contains a contradiction which may also be its undoing," he pointed out. "It is a system, based not on mutual respect but in pseudo mutuality. . . . It remains doubtful whether the shallow psychology of administrative science will really deal with the rising disaffection in American corporations. The question is whether demands will emerge within the American labor force to change the actual conditions of power which govern work. The newspeak of the facilitators attempts to keep us from this; its point is to cloak the realities of power."

It seems most likely that in some industries, and some hospitals, the intention of the new ideology of management is to cloak the realities of power, and in others the intention is to modify them, and in most cases it is probably a little of both, depending on the goals of the organization and the character of the management. Whatever their jobs, the men and women who work in hospitals are pretty much the same as their neighbors who work in offices, factories, and fields. They like to be paid, and they like to be heard, and they like to be liked, but they are not easily fooled, and where the move toward participation is only a contrivance to quiet their restlessness, they may bite back, as a psychologist quoted by Sennett from a report in *The Conference Board Record* related: "Too often we ask for employees' attitudes and opinions in great detail, but in most cases once we have the data, nothing is done with it. And this is because the employees are telling management what it doesn't want to hear, so management ignores the findings. Then they wonder why we continue to have discontent, grievances, and strikes. It would be better not to ask the employees what they believe and feel than to ask them and do nothing."

It may still be too early to tell whether the experiments reported by the HEW task force are pointing the way to a new era and whether the changes in management attitudes will endure, but 50 years after Hawthorne it shouldn't be too much to expect that those thousands of MBAs pouring out of the graduate schools into the executive corridors of Xerox, Exxon, and XYZ may have learned something valid about what makes workers work. If they have, the changes will be real, and in hospitals the time will come when doctors and nurses and others will work together and consult one another about patient care and institutional goals without (a) barking orders or (b) saluting. We're headed in that direction, and that is the end of the line.

[1] U.S. Department of Health, Education, and Welfare, Work in America: Report of a Special Task Force to the Secretary of Health Education and Welfare. Washington, DC: U.S. Government Printing Office, December 1972.

[2] Sennett, R., The Boss's New Clothes, New York Review of Books, 26:42, February 22, 1979.

[3] What Put Labor On the Defensive, Business Week, December 4, 1978, p. 56.

There Is Always Somebody on the Other Side

January 1973

In a series of meetings and conversations with health care institutional administrators and trustees, association executives, physicians, nurses and government officials, an observer got the impression during the last few weeks that the problems are mounting all over the country but the solutions, if there are any, remain for the most part out of reach, not so much for want of resources, though this certainly has to be counted among the most urgent problems, as for lack of any uniform understanding or agreement on what needs to be done—any central conviction about which way to go. For every group that was most concerned about the contradictions and frustrations of price control, for example, there was another fretting about the constraints of regional planning, and another that saw the rise of consumerism as the most threatening phenomenon, and still others considering that the obstacles would diminish, if not vanish, if only public understanding of what they were up to, and up against, could be improved.

While there were not many clear patterns of problem recognition and response that could be identified either by professional group or by region of the country, a few conclusions may be reported from these observations, always with the reservation that exceptions occur on all sides: Generally speaking, institutional administrators are more aware than others are of the impact of the rising forces of technology, regulation and public expectation and the changes these forces are bringing to traditional methods of financing, organizing and delivering health services. This is understandable, certainly, since the professionals deal mainly with the technology, and government officials at all levels for the most part are concerned with public attitudes and expectations, whereas institutional and association executives must attempt to keep all the new forces in balance, an increasingly perilous task.

Regrettably, it has to be reported that institutional trustees seemed least aware of the tempest. A hospital consultant who has current projects in work with the boards of trustees of four hospitals totaling more than 100 members suggested that less than half that many could be considered active, and not more than 10 of the trustees, in his opinion, had any real grasp of the changes that are moving hospitals into the public facility jurisdiction. A case in point was the bank president, obviously a dedicated volunteer, who complained about the laborious and time-consuming task of obtaining the necessary planning authority approvals for his hospital's multimillion dollar expansion and modernization project. "The worst of it," he fumed, "was that the people on the planning board—the so-called consumer representatives—didn't appear competent to judge anything. Who are they? What do they know?"

While it is always possible to sympathize with the view of a civic leader who is accustomed to dealing only with presidents and chairmen and doesn't comprehend that people who don't head anything may still know something, sympathy wears thin when it turn out, as it did in this case, that the approval was eventually obtained over the misgivings of the planning board, which had already approved a similar expansion project for another hospital complex in the same community and feared that overbuilding and duplication of services would result in economic and professional stagnation at some future time. As has often happened, the board lacked final authority and was incapable of standing up to the power structure, whose basic position is that opposition to expansion is "negative thinking." Except in communities that have already experienced the stagnation resulting from overexpansion a decade ago, trustees are still pointing to the benefits, or putative benefits, of competition among hospitals, apparently not understanding that competition doesn't work the same way in the market for medical services as it does in the market for shoes and shirts. There are times, to be sure, when competition produces excellence in medical services, but there are also times when it may produce disaster, and hospital trustees ought to be able to distinguish between the two more readily than they appear to do on occasion.

Another conclusion, again not surprising, is that both the administrative and professional groups in the big cities seem more aware of change, and readier to accommodate it, than do their colleagues in the smaller cities and towns—partly because the cities have had more of it, and partly also because it is the doctors in private practice who are the least affected by change, whether they think so or not, and in the cities the institutions tend to dominate the doctors, whereas in smaller communities the doctors dominate the institutions. "Our job," said the president of the board of trustees of a hospital in a two-hospital town, "is to give the doctors everything they need to do the best they can for our patients." The heads that nodded around the table were on bankers and doctors. The frowns were worn by hospital executives, who may have wished it were really that simple but knew it wasn't.

As it turned out, however, it was the smaller and not the larger institutions that seemed to be suffering most from the stringencies of price control, possibly because the larger institutions have more services, more money, and more room to hide. At any rate, it semed to be the smaller institutions in the smaller communities who moaned the most at a meeting where a Price Commission representative predicted that wage and price controls would remain in effect in the health service industry indefinitely, and it was the administrator of a small institution who was told, in reply to a question about what constituted a hardship that would justify an exception to the limitation on a price increase: "Bankruptcy."

"Well, that's a hardship," the administrator acknowledged.

It was shocking for a visitor to hear the first report of a hospital that had to borrow money to meet current expenses when it was confronted by a combination of empty beds, long-delayed Medicare payments and rejection by the Price Commission of a request for exception, but then it turned out the experience was by no means unique, and, in fact, one administrator suggested that short-term borrowing for operating as well as capital expenses would become commonplace for hospitals in the future—a circumstance whose implications became clear when an investment banker at the same meeting commented that hospital administrators don't know much about finance.

Some do, though, and an observer got the impression that those who don't, and who don't learn, may not be hospital administrators all their lives—and maybe not for many more years. There is more talk of money and mortgages, and less of medicine and management, in the informal conversation of administrators today, and the prime topic now is not any of these, actually, but what might be described as the politics of health and hospitals—the federal programs and guidelines, existing and anticipated; the state laws and regulations; the rulings and rumblings of boards and commissions and commissioners, and the strategies for dealing with all these new and rising forces.

Listening in on the conversations, which don't vary much from one section of the country to another, an observer can remark that the hospital as charitable asylum has vanished and will not be brought back by any bureaucratic or legalistic attempt to put a thumbprint on so much of what an institution spends and demand that it shall be called charity. As institutions have become medically and technologically more sophisticated, they have also become increasingly reticular business organisms, often with office, residence, parking and other retail enterprise attached or related to the medical-nursing chassis by ownership, lease, joint venture, or other arrangements as unknown to the hospitals of a few years ago as acupuncture was to the operating rooms. Seen through the thickening haze of regulation that surrounds public-interest enterprise in our time, the hospital looks about the same whether the ownership is government, community, Church or university and, in fact, the haze increasingly obscures the line—at one time an impenetrable wall—between profitmaking and nonprofit institutions. "It makes no difference whether a health provider is classified as profit-making or nonprofit," a member of the Senate Finance Committee told one hospital group, "so it doesn't really matter how health providers are classified. What does matter is how they go about their business."

How do they? As always, the method involves an overlay of organization on the cabalistic processes of medical and nursing care, a management exercise requiring an abundant fund of knowledge and an extraordinary variety of skills, foremost among which today is that of negotiation. Like the master of simultaneous chess who moves from board to board around the room making instant transitions of adversaries, situations, strategies, decisions and actions, the hospital executive moves through his succession of negotiations with patients, families, employes, doctors, trustees, community groups, insurers, bankers, planners, government officials, politicians and reporters, making arrangements and accommodations in the interest of his institution and those it serves. It is possible always for an adversary, or an interested party, or an observer of any segment or phase of any of the negotiations to find fault with the negotiator's assessment of the situation, or his strategy, or with a decision that is made, or an action that is taken, but the whole performance has to be measured comprehending the full circle of negotiations, and whoever is constrained to make a judgment had better remember that no matter where he sits there is somebody on the other side of the circle.

We'll Never Know Unless We Try

January 1979

The cost containment effort that has been the principal focus of hospital management attention for the past year and promises to continue, if not intensify, for as far ahead as anybody can see, has been directed in part toward tightening control of utilization to cut down on unnecessary services, and in part toward improving management efficiency to increase worker productivity at all levels of skill. The first goal is elusive because of the difficulties of determining medical necessity, which resides more in the minds of physicians and patients than in the data of computers. The second goal is elusive because in many hospital functions productivity is not a simple measure of volume and time related to cost but a complex measure of volume, time, cost, and quality, and the added dimension, like necessity, exists to some extent in the mind. Hospital people are accustomed to coping with these complexities, which come with the territory; cost containment, after all, did not spring unrecognized a year ago from the superior intellects of the Congress and the Department of Health, Education, and Welfare. Cost-saving methods studies have been a staple in the literature of hospital management for 50 years, and considerations of medical necessity and quality of care have been there right along, uncomprehended by the new experts hallooing down hospital corridors crying havoc.

Up to now, it has seemed likely that there is more to be saved by subtracting utilization than by adding productivity, if only somebody can figure out how to get the measure of medical necessity out of the minds and into the machines. This is what criteria and standards and utilization committees and PSROs are supposed to be doing, and are, probably as well as the state of the art permits, although nobody has been cheering wildly about the results. Nobody is cheering much, either, about the millions presumably being saved by the strictures that have been legislated and regulated into hospital and medical practice in our time for the purpose of shrinking what is seen as an over-expanded industry. A few HSAs, to be sure, have led the cheering for themselves on occasion, pointing to their rejection of this or that multi-million dollar expansion project as evidence that they have saved that much for their constituencies. But the more common experience has been one of shooting down squirrels while the lions prowl unrestrained, and the savings are more putative than real, as a family that doesn't need a car may think to save by buying a Chevrolet instead of a Cadillac. Also, HSAs at times have seen themselves as guardians of the nation's solvency when they have succeeded in closing down a few isolated obstetric departments that failed to achieve the magic number of 500 births a year, a maneuver that may make it necessary for gravid mothers to travel 50 or 100 miles to pay $1,500 for care they could have had at home for $900.

The absurdity of the approach to health planning as a numbers game was made clear a few weeks ago in the report of a study of infant mortality in a rural midwestern state where the smallest hospitals had the lowest rates.[1] The state had a system for referring high-risk cases to designated perinatal centers, established before the HSA existed, which of course accounted for the higher mortality rates at the larger centers. But the satisfactory rates and lower costs of normal deliveries at hospitals with 100 or 200 births a year reveal the costly illogic of applying factory standards to biological processes. "Review of perinatal birth and mortality statistics in Iowa for the past five years shows that small services can provide adequate perinatal care for the relatively low risk patients they serve," Herman A. Hein, M.D., principal investigator for the study, said. "The major implication of my report is that small obstetric services can offer acceptable perinatal care when they are part of a regionalized system. Perhaps the intent of the National Health Planning and Resources Development Act could be implemented more effectively by encouraging regionalized systems of perinatal care rather than by attempting to limit obstetric service size."

There can't be much doubt that closing hospital departments and hospitals in some cases saves money, but the first question is, for whom? And the next question is at what hidden cost, as for the mother who has to travel to another city, where it costs more, to have her baby—assuming she doesn't get caught in a snowdrift on the way, where it could cost more than money. The objections to planning by the numbers don't come just from trustees who fear loss of authority and administrators who fear loss of jobs and doctors who fear loss of patients, as the new gauleiters appear to believe, but mostly from people who fear loss of beds to be sick in. Those consumer members on HSA boards don't vote with the doctors because they've been conned, but because they want to keep what they have. The signals suggesting that HSAs may be expected to move from facilities planning into appropriateness review, a prospect that causes functional dyspnea among physicians and hospital administrators, are a textbook example of the bureaucratic principle that holds the thing to do with a system that isn't working is to give it something more.

A substantive element of the system that does seem to be working is the effort to encourage multi-institutional sharing and integration of services. According to one of the early actors on the multi-institutional stage, Robert Toomey of the Greenville, SC, Hospital System, 40 percent of U.S. hospitals are now participating in 400 organized management systems, and "the configuration of the nation's hospital system is changing with lightning-like rapidity."[2] Toomey described several kinds of organization, sharing and integrating many kinds of service under all kinds of arrangement, and suggested that the systems would continue to grow to include 75 percent of the industry, with a cornucopia of benefits in effectiveness of operation and improvements in services. Moreover, he said, all this is being achieved without disrupting continuity of management or autonomy for local boards of trustees of participating hospitals. As one who was practicing multiunit management 20 years ago, Toomey was generous in acknowledging that it was not the economic logic of systems management, but the advent of investor-owned chains in the 1960s, that stimulated development of the movement among voluntary hospitals, and it has been a "reaction to over-regulation by power grabbers" that has sparked the "revolutionary restructuring" now taking place. He didn't emphasize the point particularly, but unquestionably the provisions of Public Law 93-641 and the rising pressures from

HSAs have also had something to do with the current disposition of neighboring hospitals to shake hands instead of fists—a change that troubles the Federal Trade Commission as much as it pleases the Department of Health, Education, and Welfare.

It must be reported also that the cornucopia includes some rocks along with the fruit. While smaller institutions that have joined hands with larger and richer neighbors are generally relieved to have the superior technical and management resources represented in the systems, and in most cases it is likely that operating efficiencies and improvements in services have indeed resulted, there are cases of record where costs have gone up instead of down, where local boards have found themselves looking on instead of taking part, and where local physicians have discovered that there are times when their wishes are something less than law. There are also cases where administrators have involuntarily embarked on careers as consultants, and the fact that the cause in any case may have been unwillingness rather than inability to adapt to new ways of doing things doesn't make them any happier about the turn of events, or any more enthusiastic about multi-institutional management systems.

It is not especially comforting to reflect that hospitals may be following the path marked out years ago by gas stations and chain stores, and the result of a generation of change has been that 200 corporations own 60 percent of the assets of U.S. industry. We cherish the difference between hospitals and supermarkets and react with horror to the suggestion that the difference might be diminishing. But as Toomey and others have noted, the preponderance of evidence is that economy and efficiency are improved by multiunit management and that in more cases than not the systems have had the wit and the wisdom to add what is needed without subtracting what is good about local governance, and management, and patient care. And since it looks as though events are going to continue in the direction they have taken, it is up to the governors and managers and physicians of hospitals contemplating affiliation with multiunit systems to examine the proposed arrangements with a view to gaining the benefits of affiliation without sacrificing what they already have—always remembering that what they have isn't necessarily great just because it is theirs.

Whatever the organizational mode, however, or whether the

unit is shrinking or swelling, there is one promising method of saving money that is commonly overlooked, if not studiously avoided, even in this time of intense concentration on cost containment, and that is the systematic substitution of trained volunteers, family members, and patients themselves for paid staff in the performance of routine nontechnical tasks. Now wait just a minute. Professional people automatically reject the idea of working with amateurs, and administrators roll their eyes upward and pray to be spared the need to resolve arguments about jurisdiction and fears about liability. But we are supposed to be dealing here with a real crisis, where saving money is an essential for survival, not just a desirable goal to be achieved in every possible way, as long as it doesn't upset people. The experience of hospitals during strikes, power failures, floods, and other disasters has demonstrated repeatedly that volunteers and family members can provide many services ordinarily performed by staff, and that patients can do a lot of things for themselves that staff, including in some cases professional staff, consider their exclusive province.

To mention just a few of them, volunteers could serve meal trays and make beds and transport patients and run elevators and perform clerical tasks, and many of them would rather do these obviously useful jobs than the lesser ones they are commonly assigned. With just a minimum of training they could also take temperatures and blood pressures and deliver medications and keep records—and the sky would not fall, neither would the number of errors and accidents rise. The thing that would unquestionably rise would be the tempers of nurses and other professionals whose attitude toward volunteers too often is that they are unnecessary and in the way and incapable of doing any but the most superficial chores, like arranging flowers and pushing book carts. This attitude would be a formidable barrier, but it could be modified in time—if it weren't for the fact that many administrators feel exactly the same way about volunteers. The quality of care would suffer, the professionals would all insist, and since quality exists partly in the mind, who could say that they were wrong?

The same barriers would have to be surmounted to make it possible for patients and patients' families to help themselves. At the time of a critical nursing shortage some 20 years ago, a former president of the American Hospital Association proposed that a substantial fraction of hospital bed patients, with some help from members of their families, might be encouraged to get their own meals, keep their own records, move themselves to diagnostic and therapeutic departments as indicated, and take their own medications—as they did anyway, necessarily, from the moment they left the hospital. If patients can be trusted to take the right medicine at the right time the day after they leave the hospital, he asked, why can't they do it the day before? The proposal was made in a serious paper presented at a professional meeting, and the reaction to it—at the time and afterward—was silent contemplation of their fingernails by the author's professional colleagues.

It seems likely that the professional reaction would be the same today, when it would also be pointed out that in many institutions there would be violent opposition to assigning volunteers and families to duties customarily performed by nurses, aides, orderlies, and others belonging to unions. It would be argued, too, that the cost of recruiting and training volunteers for these tasks, and scheduling the work, and supervising patients and families, would be an offset against savings, which wouldn't be all that great anyway. But we'd never know until we tried it, and if the Congress were as serious as it says it is about hospital costs it could pass an amendment to the labor relations act making it possible for hospitals to substitute volunteers for union members in the interest of cost containment.

The substitution won't be undertaken seriously by hospitals, however, and even if it were the Congress wouldn't risk upsetting labor by considering any such legislation. Because the fact is that while we are all earnest and sincere about the cost containment effort, earnestness and sincerity are not to be pushed beyond the borders of accepted attitudes and practices and jurisdictions, either in the professions or in government. The cost crisis is a real crisis, all right, but not that real.

[1] Hein, L.A., The Quality of Perinatal Care in Small Rural Hospitals, Journal American Medical Association, 20:2070, November 3, 1978.

[2] Toomey, R., Multi-hospital Systems, presented to the First National Symposium on the Hospital Market, conducted by Hospitals and Trustee, Chicago: October 30-31, 1978.

Who's Minding
the Store?

March 1978

As pundits inside and outside the health care culture indulge
in the popular indoor sport of enumerating the alleged excesses
and deficiencies of hospitals, it is commonly assumed that hospital trustees uniformly are either unaware that their supposed
derelictions exist or unequipped to deal with them decisively.
Now unqualified assertions about hospital trustees, as about
most species, are more likely than not to be wrong on the face of
it, but it is probably true that there are a few members of many
hospital boards, and many members of a few boards, who have
remained largely unaware of the extent to which changes in the
professional, social, and political environment have influenced
the scope of their decision-making authority and the impact of
their decisions. The trustees one encounters at hospital association meetings and educational conferences, like teetotalers at a
temperance lecture, are inclined to be those least in need of the
treatment being dispensed, but they at least seem generally to
understand that the terms of the assignment are changing. If
anything, however, they may tend to be misled by the intimidating masses of detail thrown about on these occasions and to
overestimate the degree to which their authority has been
invaded—sometimes to the point where they seem to need re-
minding that they are still running the place.

In fact, the most significant result of all the environmental
changes may be that governing boards really are running the
place today, and not simply making certain that there is money
enough for their administrators to get the doctors everything
they need, or think they need. To a large extent, the patient care
decisions made by physicians still determine how hospital resources are used, and always will, but the rising external pressures of recent years have made it necessary for boards to assert
the authority they have always had, but used only rarely in the

250

past, to insist that the limits on resources and conditions of use are observed, and not just formulated and forgotten. The forces of economics, technology, law, regulation, and consumerism are compelling the hospital to behave like a corporate entity, as it has always appeared to outsiders to be, much as it may remain a federation of independent duchies in the eyes of dukes. Surprisingly under the circumstances, the incidence of collision of medical and lay authority does not appear to have increased markedly. It may be that the doctors' automatic outrage at the imposition of limits and conditions of practice is muted within the sheltering corporate arms of the hospital, where the fierce winds of circumstance are scarcely felt by physicians. Up to now, at least, nobody has proposed a 9 percent limit on annual increases in their fees.

However it came about, there can be little doubt that the sharp lines dividing the hospital into discrete jurisdictions of board, medical staff, and administration have been blurring, as physicians are appointed to boards and board committees and take an increasingly active part in corporate activities, and as board members and administrators, spurred by court decisions moving toward corporate responsibility, keep closer watch on medical affairs and, especially, medical results. The board member or administrator who a short time ago wouldn't have known a cholecystectomy from a collarbone may go to a board or committee meeting today with a computer printout in his pocket and a sharp question about a vagrant diagnostic statistic in his mind. He'll ask his question and get an answer, because everybody in the room knows that the next person to ask the same question could be in a government or insurance company office, or in court.

It doesn't make much sense, though, to consider that every trustee has to be knowledgeable about the evaluation of medical performance. Given the outside pressures, every hospital board has to have a few members, at least, who understand the system and know what the figures mean, and these members shouldn't all be doctors. There should also be a few who are on the way to becoming knowledgeable, and that doesn't happen overnight, and the rest of the members need to know enough to understand what the others are talking about and back up their decisions. In this age of specialization, there can't be anything wrong with having some trustees who concentrate on medical evaluation, and some on finance, and some on management, and some planning—as long as they're all involved in something and are willing to listen to one another and make decisions. A difficulty with education programs for hospital trustees has been that many of them are aimed at teaching everything to everybody; it's as though every doctor on the staff had to know everything from pediatrics to neurosurgery. The trustee who knows he doesn't have time to learn everything may often be turned off before he learns anything.

The thing that all policymakers do need to understand is the way centers of decision-making control have been shifting. This is what has been happening in all areas of governance responsibility—medicine, money, management, planning, and public policy. Thus in medicine the control remains with the individual physician where the care of his patients is concerned, but for consideration of patient care as a collective phenomenon the focus is enlarged from the medical staff organization to the corporate institution—and beyond, as Professional Standards Review Organizations either review or supervise review of Medicare and Medicaid patient care. This is a matter of corporate concern: An organizational instrument of the federal government can make decisions determining whether or not the hospital shall be paid for the care of a significant number of its patients. The existence of such external decision-making authority may create occasions where the institution's collective responsibility for patient care impinges on the physician's distributive responsibility. As a practical matter, hospital decisions have not been seriously invaded by PSROs, so the effect is limited, but awareness that a measure of control has slipped away may influence decisions on hospital activities. The medical staff organization that is performing its review and evaluation tasks conscientiously and capably is least likely to encourage attention from outside the walls. It may be that lawsuits and PSRO have done more in the past two or three years to awaken hospitals to the need for quality control than 50 years of hospital standardization and accreditation have done—a possibility that must cause wakeful nights among thoughtful believers in the voluntary way.

There can't be many hospital trustees or administrators or physicians of sound mind and unimpaired ability to read and hear and count who are not familiar with the extent to which control of its own financial affairs has shifted outside the hospital—to insurers, unions, government agencies, and rate review boards, as well as to banks, bond houses, and other sources of capital in the money market. But there may be many who are not aware of the potential for further inroads, not to say raids, on hospital financial autonomy. Medicare reimbursement may come close to reaching the cost of Medicare services but still subtract something from hospital control, and Medicaid reimbursement may be influenced more by the condition of state solvency than by the content of Medicaid services, and subtract something more from control. State hospital commissions already are reviewing budgets or rates in some jurisdictions, and it seems inevitable that the practice will spread to others. On the principle that it is generally easier to keep an eye on the statehouse than it is on the White House, state commissions are regarded as a lesser malady than federal bureaus, whose guidelines have a way of becoming commandments, and the hospital commission may actually be desirable in states where reimbursement rates are now being reviewed by insurance departments or health departments, and where hospitals can obtain adequate representation on the commissions. But it could be a disaster where the commissioners are political appointees less interested in hospitals than in headlines. There may be no way to keep this from happening, the way things are, but the best preventive measure may be for hospital trustees to mobilize and deploy their considerable influence in the interest of constructive legislative action in the states.

Nobody needs to be reminded of the way law and regulation have hemmed in hospital planning decisions, which must now comprehend not just the institution's own objectives for the future but those of all the other health care institutions and programs in the area. Hospital representatives who have been active in planning are now familiar with the frustrations of dealing with Health Systems Agencies whose life and death power over plans for facilities and services is exercised by HSA boards that are (a) controlled by consumer majorities, and (b) just learning their business, and (c) under federal mandate, soon to be enshrined in guidelines, to cut down the number of hospital beds in the country and keep expenditures for new equipment at the absolute minimum consistent with avoiding rioting in the streets. Here again, the cue for hospital boards is not that they must master all the demographic characteristics of the population, the rates of use of all the hospital beds and instruments, the numbers and ages of all the physicians in all the specialties, the space allocations for all the functions of all the hospitals, and the desires of all the consumer organizations and neighborhood Naders, whose crotchets often spring forth unexpectedly in accusatory headlines. These phenomena are grist for the mills of professional planners. But the boards need to be sure that their planners are on the job and know what they're doing, because the hospital trustees and executives will be called on to make decisions and spend money based on planning recommendations. And their plans will be subjected to increasingly severe scrutiny by HSA watchdogs, and watchdogs of watchdogs, as time goes by.

For years, hospital administrators and trustees have worried, sometimes together and sometimes separately, about the proper assignment of functions to their respective jurisdictions. What are management's tasks and decisions, and what are the board's? More often than not, the issues were resolved with solemn declarations that the board is responsible for policy and the management for operations. This satisfied everybody and worked well enough in matters where policies were established in existing practice and routines for conducting operations were in place, but the question kept coming up as practices changed and new functions were created. Moreover, there were always areas where policy shaded into operations and operations shaded into policy, and it was hard to tell which was which.

As it has turned out, however, at a time when the pace of change is furious and new problems come up every day, if not every hour, the question is rarely heard, probably not so much because it has been resolved as because the pressures have obscured the old boundary lines here too, and it has become obvious that there are times when the administration must take the initiative in policy matters and times when the board had better dig into operations and help administration solve problems. And if everybody stood around worrying still about who did what, the policies would never be established and the problems would never be solved. Meanwhile, there are standards by which management performance can be evaluated in hospitals, as there are in most businesses. Because of the obvious difference in mission, hospital standards are not the same as those of other businesses, but they are not all that different, either. Trustees need to know both the differences and the similarities in order to make judgments and know where their hospitals stand, so they can avoid wasting time on details and raise questions only when performance appears to be out of line. When it is, they want to be asking the questions themselves, before somebody out there in a PSRO, HSA, or some other office or agency asks them.

That isn't as farfetched as it sounds, and it isn't necessarily wrong. Almost half the money paid to hospitals now comes form tax sources. In obedience to a political canon that has been observed at least since Caesar conquered all Gaul, responsibility goes where the money comes from, so public policy requires that there should be some public effort to safeguard against unnecessary expense. We can, and do, object to public regulation that is unreasonable, or ineffective, or misapplied, or needlessly costly. But those who object to regulation *qua* regulation, as many still do, probably should not accept assignment as hospital trustees except in institutions that have no public patients. Elsewhere, hospital governance is in part a public responsibility, and not less so because the hospital may be an unwilling partner to the public contract. Like them or not, those are *our* watchdogs.

It seems clear that the Congress wants to keep hospitals in the role of supplier, not servant. Nearly 10 years elapsed between enactment of the major entitlements and the hard bite of regulation on utilization and cost, which came only after it was plain that voluntary controls, such as they were, weren't working. Even now, the Congress has seemed willing to back off the proposal to crack down on hospital revenues and give industry control another chance, which can work only if individual hospital boards and administrations and physicians prove willing to give up another measure of their own internal control in the interest of social policy. For some, this may mean giving up beds and services, as well as another slice of autonomy, and it will test whether the health care industry is strong enough to do what John Stuart Mill, the British utilitarian philosopher, insisted "is never done nor expected to be done, save in very exceptional cases, by any depositaries of power—namely, to direct their conduct by their real ultimate interest, in opposition to their immediate and apparent interest." It seems plain that the real ultimate interest of hospitals is to retain decisions about beds and services and revenues within the industry to the greatest possible extent, and this is a goal that can be achieved only at the sacrifice of the immediate and apparent interest of the institutions that have to give something up. The interests of physicians are caught up in the same tensions, and it is not clear whether or how these are going to be resolved.

The ultimate and immediate interests of hospitals may be in opposition soon in another context as government and industry, as well as some leaders of medical and hospital thought, have become convinced that effective control of excessive demand for health care services requires new emphasis on preventive measures and, especially, on motivating people to take a greater share of responsibility for their own health, and teaching them how. Unquestionably with an eye on its bills for employees' health insurance, industry is taking a new interest in helping its people keep well, with activities ranging from breathing exercises at desks and workbenches to classes for those who want to quit smoking and counsel for overeaters and drinkers. But doctors and hospitals, to whom the rest of us look for leadership in everything having anything to do with health, will have to join and sustain these efforts if they are to have any lasting effect on the health status of the population. Many hospitals have initiated new programs of public health education in recent months, but it remains to be seen whether this is acceptance of a new community responsibility or just another fad that will enjoy its vogue as a topic for conference programs, and then vanish. These are matters for sober thought among hospital policymakers. Is the mission here to make a positive contribution to the health of the population, or is it basically to find a body for every bed? The events that flow from this policy decision by the nation's hospitals will have a lot to do with the direction in which control of hospital activities may move in the future.

Educating Trustees:
Redefining the Process

November 1976[1]

The terms of this assignment, redefining the process of educating trustees, suggest that the process has already been defined somewhere, by somebody, and, if that is the case, then it turns out that I am behind with my homework again, because I have been paddling around, or at any rate treading water, in the pool of trustee education for a year or more now, and dipping my toe into the water off and on for some 30 years without ever encountering anything that looked very much like a definition. It may also be mission impossible, because what is right for A may be poison for B.

So I am making my own rules here, and I am going to begin by describing one example of the process of trustee education that is familiar to me, and I suppose also to some of you. This is a published report of a conference that was planned for the education of hospital trustees:

> In a meeting punctuated by lively exchanges between the panel and the audience, trustees from half a dozen hospitals held a mock board meeting, then answered questions from an audience of hospital trustees about their deliberations and decisions. The questions were directed to board members, sometimes with considerable top-spin, by the moderator—a member of the board of a New York City hospital. The session began with a sober presentation on trustee responsibilities by the president of the board of a New Jersey medical center, who got the audience of administrators and trustees on his side right away be declaring that if trustees gave their full time to the job, well-trained administrators would either go crazy or have no time left to perform their own duties. The speaker also cast his vote for small (15 member) boards, slow turnover of board members, complete authority for the administrator, board responsibility for patient care, generous use of hospital consultants, patient opinion surveys, modern management methods, regional integration of hospital facilities, and a firm answer for hospital critics.

> When the speaker finished, the mock board meeting got underway. The

administrator (this role was played by an administrator, not a trustee) reported that a study made by the personnel policies committee of the fictional hospital had revealed that doctors and nurses weren't getting along at all well together, a circumstance that evoked a sympathetic titter from the audience. However, the administrator added, things were looking up: A new personnel manager had been employed, some meetings were being held with department heads, and attitudes were improving. A board member wanted to know if this meant that the trustees on the personnel committee were getting mixed up in administrative functions. The administrator acknowledged that this possibility made him nervous at the beginning, but it hadn't worked out that way. The board dealt with policy and left practice up to him, he explained, as heads nodded all around the room. He didn't mention how to tell the difference. From here on there was less sweetness and light. A woman board member read a letter from the president of the auxiliary to the president of the board suggesting some kind of fund raising activity. In the discussion that followed she suggested that the auxiliary should be represented on the board so the women would know what the boys in the back room were thinking. This caused trouble. One board member took a dim view of what he called the "nibbling approach" to fund raising. Another member felt that money should be welcomed in any quantity, but he thought the board should keep posted on what the auxiliary was doing and have authority to approve or disapprove their projects in advance. Somebody else wanted to know why the auxiliary's letter had been addressed to the president of the board instead of the administrator. The woman member wanted to know, "Why not?" Discussion of this question revealed that opinion was divided as to whether or not the shortest distance from the auxiliary to the board is a straight line through the administrator. The administrator said absolutely, and the woman member said absolutely not. There was disagreement, too, about auxiliary representation on the board, but general agreement that there should be some means of keeping the board informed about auxiliary projects. And, somebody suggested, vice versa. There was no dissent.

On this happy note, the discussion moved along to consider an application for staff membership from a doctor who was obviously, on the face of it, a professional genius and a copper-riveted stinker. The application had come along by the prescribed route—credentials committee of the staff through the executive committee of the staff to the joint conference committee to the board. To apprehensive board members who wanted to take another look before approving the application, the chairman of the joint conference committee replied that the committee had already investigated reports that the applicant, as a member of the hospital's courtesy staff, had had trouble with the obstetrical supervisor, or vice versa. "I'd rather lose a doctor than an OB supervisor," the administrator groaned. When the laughter died down, he added that with the cooperation of the chief of the department he was sure that the applicant would become, as the joint conference committee had euphemistically expressed it, "a cooperative member of the hospital family." When it came to a vote, however, the board decided to consider the matter further, and put the decision off until its next meeting.

The next question was money. The treasurer reported gloomily that the hospital's financial position had been getting steadily more unfavorable—a statement that evoked laughter in the audience, but with overtones of hysteria. Losses were going up, and rates would have to be increased, the treasurer recommended. Some members wanted an across the board increase in room rates; others thought service charges should be increased selectively in accordance with rising costs. The board member who raised the question about the auxiliary said that if the hospital had a gift shop, as had been suggested repeatedly, maybe they wouldn't have to raise rates. The men were patient and polite but were obviously thinking about the many differences between a gift shop and a gold mine. Eventually the meeting arrived at a species of consensus: Rates are a public concern; rate decisions should be made only after full consideration of reliable public relations information and advice, and this should be taken up by the board—next month.

That ended the mock board meeting. In the question and answer period that followed it may be significant that the only issues that were raised and discussed—heatedly and at length—had not been mentioned at the meeting. These were: whether or not department heads should attend board meetings, and whether or not doctors on the staff should be elected to the board.

As I suspect you may have deduced by this time, this exercise in trustee education is not exactly current. In fact, this account appeared in the October 1952 issue of a hospital journal, in a report of the 1952 convention of the American Hospital Association in Philadelphia, which included this session for trustees. While it developed that there were some trustees in the audience, as well as on the program, the majority of those attending were administrators. Some things don't change that much over the years.

A lot of things obviously have changed, however, and perhaps a review of these may give us some clues about the extent to which the processes of trustee education have been redefined by circumstance. For example, there was no mention anywhere of planning in the 1952 session; if there had been, it would have been a concern for the building fund drive, or with some detail of space allocation or construction cost for a proposed new building. In any comparable board meeting or education session today planning would surely be a central concern, and the possible considerations would range from terms and interest rates on a major borrowing to the strategy of obtaining planning board approval of a proposed equipment installation and the need to push discussions with a neighboring hospital about consolidation of pediatric departments. If the matter of space allocations for a new building were a hospital problem, it would have been handed down the line and probably settled at the second level of management.

Administrators and board members of my generation—and a few of us are still animate—may remember when it was possible for trustees to argue about how, and how much, rates should be raised, but it is unlikely that the trustee at the 1952 meeting had any idea how prophetic he was when he said that rates are a public concern. Moreover, it seems likely, if not inevitable, that hospital people a few years from now will look back at 1976 as a time when they still had something to say about how much they would be paid for some of their services, by some of their funding sources.

In redefining the process of trustee education it must certainly be noted that all these issues of planning and building and equipment and rates have to be, or should be, examined today in relation to definitions of hospital mission—as determined by the board, still, but not without a certain amount of assistance from external sources. There was no mention of mission in 1952. There was no mention, either, of another subject that would certainly be at center stage at any board meeting or education conference today—quality assurance. Incidentally, too, any alert board today would be a lot more cautious about how they discussed considerations of personality difficulties with an applicant for staff membership, who would certainly sue the hospital and the officers and perhaps members of its board of trustees and medical staff if his application were turned down, and might readily sue if it were only delayed. Another notable difference between then and now, not totally unrelated to the redefinition of trustee education, is that today the Cadillacs in the hospital parking lot belong to the lawyers, not the surgeons. The chauffered limousine at the front door belongs to a union organizer.

This recitation might run on through the entire litany of hospital interests and affairs, and I expect in most cases the contrasts would be as sharp as the ones I have mentioned here. So it may be comforting to note one or two things that have not changed much, if at all. One is the insistence that the board of trustees is concerned with policy and the management with operations, and the reason we don't explain exactly what that means is the same now as it was then. We don't know. The closest I can come to a definition is that if it is $5,000, it's operations, and if it's $50,000, it's policy.

Another thing that is still being argued is doctors on the board, but the argument is more theoretical than it used to be, because it turns out that about half the hospitals already have doctors on the board, and as far as I know none of the dreadful problems that were supposed to follow on this breach of what was once seen as proper practice have occurred. The answer being, I expect, that some doctors, like some lawyers and bankers and storekeepers and farmers and school teachers, are capable of putting self-interest aside and devoting their intelligence and their energies to the betterment of their communities, and some aren't. I don't think we can fairly or reasonably assume that *all* physician trustees are pursuing private goals of their own for their own gain. With careful consideration, and perhaps a little bit of luck, it should be possible in most cases to pick doctors who will make good trustees, but I should think the board would wish to retain the responsibility for doing the picking, and not delegate it to the medical staff. They might be looking for different things.

Given the difference of time and circumstance, we might consider for a moment whether or not the mock board meeting at the 1952 AHA convention was good trustee education. Certainly it was lively and interesting for its audience, and was even entertaining at times, and I don't think any of those qualities should be ignored as irrelevant. Sober pedagogical research has established that students learn more from a teacher whom they consider to be entertaining than from one they consider to be dull, and, in fact, this has been demonstrated at the reasonably advanced intellectual level of first and second year medical school classes. I suppose it can be argued, too, that almost any discussion of current topics—even though the topics in this case may seem unbelievably simple-minded to us now from the distance of 24 years—is of itself educational. But I think this is true only if the discussion goes to the reasons for things and examines the principles underlying opinions that are expressed and decisions and actions that are taken. That wasn't done in this case, at least it doesn't appear in the account we have here, and I don't remember that it happened at the meeting itself, which I attended as a reporter.

So what was learned, actually? It is possible, I suppose, that some administrators and trustees in the 1952 audience may have been enlightened to discover that trustees who monkey around in operations are not universally applauded for their efforts, and some may have been surprised at the time that trustees consider it their proper business to question a medical staff recommendation on credentials, and that decisions about rates might be considered a legitimate interest of some who don't have access to hospital board rooms and country club locker rooms. These were important lessons then, and I expect there are places, though I hope not many, where they might still be important lessons today, and I am not inclined to belittle them. But education as we are talking about it here, I should think, must comprehend something more than bringing the word to backward nations, so to speak, and certainly there were educational opportunities in that session that were unrecognized, questions unasked, and principles unsought for. If somebody had asked, for example, *why* the board was looking at credentials, and the reasons had been examined and the implications considered and the principle established, it is possible, at least, that it wouldn't have taken us 20 years to get to the point where quality assurance is a widely accepted board responsibility, and we might not have had it shoved down our throats in a court decision in 1965 and then in an amendment to the Social Security Act in 1972. If somebody back there in 1952 had picked up the proposition that hospital rates are a public concern, and we had all looked at it thoughtfully and carefully and studied its implications and formulated the basic principle, then we might not have state rate commissions and HSAs telling us what we can and can't do. We might have organized our own classification systems and prospective budgeting plans instead of having them laid on us by law and administrative fiat. Nobody can be *sure* these things wouldn't have happened anyway, of course, but I think we can agree that the education of 25 years ago was superficial, at best, and maybe there is a message here as we consider what we want our trustees to know about, and think about, today. Maybe that is what we are doing at this conference.

[1]Adapted from an address to a forum on educating hospital trustees sponsored by the W.K. Kellogg Foundation, Memphis, TN: November 1976.

It's Not That Kind of Job

October 1979

A dozen or so years ago we all started talking about "health care," a term which is imprecise but was useful for Medicare and other services that were plainly not comprehended in "medical care" or "hospital care," which had served nicely up to that time. Over the same years we have also referred freely to the "health professions," or sometimes the "allied health professions," using these terms, again, as though we knew just what we were talking about. Actually we don't. "Health professions" most of the time probably refers to physicians and nurses and all the old and new subdoctors and subnurses and technicians and others who help doctors and nurses find out what's wrong and then do something about it. "Allied professions" obviously are all the others except doctors and nurses, who have staked out their own territories in the terminology.

Now the dictionary says it is accurate and proper to refer to any distinctive occupation as a profession, as we do right along when we talk about professional ball players, for example, or the insurance profession, as some say, or, on occasion, the world's oldest profession. But that isn't what we mean when we refer to the allied health professions, because we wouldn't consider the term to include hospital orderlies or maids or maintenance men, even though these are professions in the occupational sense and are more related to health than, say, English teachers, who certainly do belong to a profession, though it would appear to be one of diminishing influence.

The other dictionary meaning of profession is the one to which the modifier "learned" is either applied or implied, and it is commonly used to identify doctors, lawyers, teachers, and clergy. This was a practice that had its origin at a time when these were the only people around who had been to college and knew Greek and history and could play the violin, and it persists even today, when the colleges teach computers instead of history and most doctors haven't had time to learn English, let alone Greek. Use of the modifier, spoken or implied, is still restricted to these professions, unscholarly as many of their practitioners may have become. But while the modifier is never used nor intended elsewhere, we often describe architecture and engineering, for example, as professions in other than the occupational or livelihood meaning, and we invariably do so with nursing. In these professions that are almost learned professions there are telltale signs that the "almost" grates, as when architects or nurses make a point of insisting that theirs *are* professions, in tones meaning that they *are too* professions—as though anybody else ever gave it a thought. Engineers do the same thing. They have a National *Professional* Engineering Society; the adjective is probably intended to distinguish the ones who build bridges and skyscrapers from those who run trains and boilers, but it has a certain anxiety quotient nevertheless. Again, as though anybody else cared. But we make unconscious distinctions. Thus we never refer to the corporation president as professional, though he may be more learned in any instance than the professor of internal medicine, and the Ph.D. in molecular biology is a professional if he is on a medical school faculty, but not if he is in a pharmaceutical company laboratory. The logic is obscure, but traces of it that become visible on examination suggest that the usage is not entirely whimsical.

The characteristics of the learned professions are well known and have been written about at least since Plato's time. The profession has a discrete body of knowledge requiring long and intensive preparation, including instruction in skills and methods as well as in the scientific, historical, or scholarly principles underlying them. The body of knowledge of the learned profession is primarily intellectual in nature. There is a body of knowledge to be mastered in learning auto mechanics, for example, but auto mechanics is not therefore regarded as a profession except in the occupational sense. In the learned professions, access is formalized and disciplined; there are no side doors or back doors, and entry into the practice of the professional skills and methods is barred to outsiders by public policy as in laws requiring licensure, registration, or certification and penalizing practice by the unqualified. The profession has known standards of achievement and methods of dealing with failure to meet them; courts recognize such failure as a proper cause for action by those who may be damaged. Finally, the profession has known standards of conduct, or ethics, committing its members to the pursuit of knowledge and performance the primary purpose of which is human betterment or public service, not private gain, with a system for disciplining the errant.

Plainly by these standards medicine and law and teaching and the ministry meet most of the requirements, though the bodies of knowledge for teaching and the ministry are thin for some members, exclusivity is often weak, and high standards of performance and conduct inconsistently applied. But inconsistency of performance doesn't rule a profession out of consideration, or we shouldn't have any; medicine and law qualify historically and currently on all counts, which is not to say that doctors uniformly invoke sanctions disciplining their poor performers and bad actors, or that lawyers are all that eager for human betterment regardless of the size of the fee. Ask any client.

So what about the health professions? Nursing historically has the name and standing as a profession and, all things considered, probably comes closer to being truly professional than the others commonly subsumed as "allied"—presumably meaning allied to medicine. But nursing has inconsistencies of its own. You can't call three years after high school long and intensive preparation, for example, and while a lot of the body of nursing knowledge is properly scientific and intellectual, a lot of it isn't. Nevertheless, entry into the profession is formalized, and practice is limited by public policy and force of law. Nursing gets mixed scores on standards of performance and conduct, because more often than not these are imposed from outside the profession by physicians and hospitals rather than inside by professional consensus. But it should be noted that standards of performance may also be imposed on nurses by conditions of employment not of their own choosing. And nursing gets high marks for the pursuit of knowledge; the emphasis on baccalaureate and graduate programs in recent years has to be considered a step up on the ladder of professionalism, although there are those who say it may not do much for human betterment if it tends to put nurses in offices instead of in patients' rooms. The human betterment score is clouded anyway by nurses' strikes on economic issues, and not notably improved by the fact that the strikes may do a lot for the human betterment of nurses themselves, or by the argument that this may be better for patients in the end. A strike may be justified in any given case, but nobody is going to call it professional. Nurses and doctors who strike may win on the issues, but they lose, incalculably, in the public respect for the professions.

The rest of the health professions can be measured by the same value system and placed closer or farther away from the learned professions, according to how they are viewed on the size and nature of the body of knowledge, method of preparation, access or entry, public policy, standards of performance and conduct, and dedication to human betterment. For purposes of this discussion, dentistry and osteopathy can be considered as branches of medicine, though some physicians would blanch at the branch. Many physicians feel much the same way about chiropody, and the issue is hot in one or two states where chiropodists want hospital privileges and doctors insist that they shall not pass, not because of any animosity but because they don't measure up as equals on the professional scales, however much they may be needed and appreciated by the patients who call them "doctor." A special case of a different kind is psychology, which is closely allied to medicine at times, as when well-trained psychologists and physicians may share respect and exchange referrals, and utterly unallied at other times, when half-educated psychologists may hang out shingles and offer counseling to troubled but unwary souls who have no way of knowing the difference. And that is what is unprofessional about psychology. The body of knowledge is scholarly and extensive, if not always rigorously scientific, but entry and access are unguarded by either public policy or effective professional consensus. Standards of performance and conduct are observed only by the elite for the elite, and with all its vast potential for human betterment, psychology has a way to go to achieve true professional status.

The other professions or subprofessions allied in one way or another with medicine—the medical laboratory, radiology, and operating room technicians, dietitians, practical nurses and nurse's aides, occupational therapists and physical therapists and inhalation therapists, and all the others—can be judged in the same way by anybody who is familiar, as hospital administrators have to be, with their levels and methods of preparation and qualification and their standards of performance and conduct. The Veterans Administration reportedly has listed more than 200 distinct hospital occupations, and the chances are that most of them consider themselves allied health professions. But some of them have well-established routes of entry and certification procedures and some haven't; some have bodies of knowledge that have to be learned, some have only skills, and some haven't much of either. Some are dedicated to patient care and some wouldn't know a patient if they saw one out of bed, and thus have to be considered less professional than the others in this respect. And here is a dimension of the professions that has to be evaluated along with knowledge and preparation and standards and conduct. The physical therapist, for example, works directly with patients all the time, and any physical therapy patient can tell you that the personal relationship is central to the effectiveness of the treatment. Is the therapist therefore more professional than the laboratory technician, for whom the patient is simply an abstraction represented by samples and cells?

Public policy and common sense suggest that the answer has to be yes. The doctor-patient and lawyer-client and teacher-pupil and priest-communicant relationships are all recognized in law. The nurse-patient relationship, bonded by touching, is unquestionably the reason nursing attained the status of profession long before its educational and performance requirements began to be elevated. The well-known sensitivity of pathologists and radiologists owes something to the fact that they never peer down throats or prod abdomens; they consider themselves as professional as other doctors are, but they are aware that nobody else quite does, and it rankles. Historically, writers about the professions almost without exception have mentioned the personal service component, and so it has to take its place here as we estimate the professional standing of social service workers, say, compared to radiology technicans, or, for that matter, psychologists compared to corporate tax consultants. It doesn't mean that one is more professional than the other, but it is something that has to be put on the scales and weighed along with everything else.

What about hospital administration, or, as some would have it now, health administration? Administrators, or those who think about it at all, are inclined to think of themselves as professional in more than the occupational sense. Their juxtaposition to medicine makes them understandably sensitive on the subject, and the fact that nobody else cares one way or the other adds to the sensitivity. While it would seem to be a minor concern at a time when hospitals are beleaguered by problems of cost, regulation, occupancy, energy, technology, and a few million others, it keeps coming up, and it may be instructive to apply the measurements that have been used by others, and reviewed here, to see where hospital administration comes out.

There is a body of knowledge of hospital administration, to be sure, but it is not discrete and it will be less so if the focus of the profession and the practice is going to be enlarged to include the administration of all kinds of institutions and programs having to do with health, a gallimaufry that might be expected to admit everybody from deans of medicine to promoters for weight watching programs. For hospital administrators, the body of knowledge is both intellectual and experiential, and a large part of it is borrowed—a little from medicine and public health, some from history and from economics, and statistics, and psychology, and public administration, and business management, which itself is a pastiche of borrowings but whose graduates don't have to worry about whether or not they are seen as professionals, or whether or not they really are. The preparation of hospital administrators is more rigorous than that of many teachers and ministers, depending on the disciplines and the levels, but less so than that of doctors and lawyers. The mode of entry into the practice of hospital administration is becoming more and more formalized, but there are still side doors and back doors that are ajar, and again, if we consider the profession to be health rather than hospital administration it won't do much good to bar the doors because there won't be any walls.

This matter of barring the doors to the unqualified is important, because public policy is involved. The professions are clothed with public interest; licensure and registration are considered necessary to protect those who receive professional services from the harm that could be done by unprepared practitioners. Up to now no such need has been perceived in the case of hospital administrators, and the management of medical institutions is sufficiently removed from the practice of medicine that it might be difficult to demonstrate a danger except perhaps to the balance sheet, or in the rare instance when an administrator may act to prevent damage by an incompetent or unethical physician because the medical profession's apparatus has failed. Hospital administration itself has standards of performance and a professional society that recognizes achievement, but poor performers are called to account by employers rather than by peer pressure. The society has a code of ethical conduct for its members, which is commendable. But the purpose of having standards of ethical conduct in the professions is to safeguard the patients and clients—those who receive the professional services—from being harmed by unethical or immoral conduct, and the position of hospital administrators as managers of institutions whose policies are established and controlled not by the managers, but by governing bodies employing the managers, means that the code of ethics of the professional society of hospital administrators can have only limited relevance to the public interest.

Finally, if we are to consider, as many do, that the personal relationship with and service to its patients or clients or pupils is an essential component of a profession, administration by its very nature—directing the efforts of others toward the achievement of a goal—is excluded from the primary rank of the professions that have all the generally recognized attributes, and must be ranked instead as an "almost learned" profession, though certainly on balance foremost among those that are called allied. It should be plain to anybody, and most of all to hospital administrators, that this view does not in any way diminish the stature, or the importance to the public, of hospital administration, nor does it mean that the individual hospital administrator is in any way a lesser person than the physician, any more than the stature or importance of a corporation president is diminished because he is not a senator. They serve the society in different ways, and it happens that the activities and functions of the corporation president and the hospital administrator are less publicly visible than those of the senator and physician, but not therefore less valuable. If it is visibility and public appreciation that the hospital administrator who longs for recognition as a professional, like the physician, is seeking, he isn't going to get it by making speeches and sending out news releases. He isn't going to get it at all, because it isn't that kind of job or that kind of profession, and if that is what he wants, the thing for him to do is quit his job and go to medical school.

Q: Who's In Charge?
A: Of What?

March 1980

A well-known and respected hospital executive likes to tell about an experience he had many years ago as a young administrator. He was up on one of the patients' floors talking to the nurse in charge when an impressively dressed matron burst into the corridor from a patient's room a few doors from where they were standing. Obviously agitated about something, she accosted a resident who happened to be passing. "I've got to see the manager!" she demanded. "Who runs this hospital, anyway?"

The resident raised both hands and rolled his eyes toward the ceiling. "Absolutely nobody, Madam," he said. "Absolutely nobody."

The question is not infrequent, and an administrator who thinks the answer in this case was entertaining and tells it on himself can probably be considered more secure than one who would be embarrassed or upset by it. All it means, actually, is that the relationship of the hospital and the doctors is unique and complicated and understood only dimly by a lot of physicians. It is also understood only dimly by a lot of hospital trustees, and not understood at all by outsiders—certainly not by the lawmakers and rule makers who keep trying to change physician behavior by putting handcuffs on hospitals.

So there is some exaggeration in the assertion of another respected administrator who says the question is dumb to begin with and is also a sure sign that hospital-physician relationships in an institution are not what they should be and it will take more than an answer to get them straightened out. This is the proposition of a lively new book for hospital trustees and administrators by Robert R. Cadmus, M.D., who knows that the question is innocent of any such sinister meaning except when it is asked, with angry sarcasm, by a physician who doesn't

270

expect an answer anyway.[1] According to Cadmus, a physician who has been a hospital administrator and president of a medical college and is now directing a foundation for medical care, the problem is that some physicians, and some trustees and administrators, don't always understand the difference between the practice of medicine and the provision of medical care, or, put another way, the difference between taking care of patients and running the place. It's when they jump their fences that they get in each others' way. Administrators never jump twice, Cadmus says, because they get fired the first time. There are some trustees who meddle with medicine, and everything else, but the most common trespasser is the physician who thinks only doctors should have anything to do with anything doctors have anything to do with, and wants to do everything himself.

Getting along with this kind of doctor is like taming lions, says Cadmus, who is not above indulging in a bit of hyperbole. "You've got to do something, but what?" he suggests. "If you overreact, if you whip the lion or poke at it needlessly, it may well roll over. But beware. It will be watching every move you make, looking for a chance to get even. If, on the other hand, you enter the cage unsure of yourself, lose the lion's attention, or permit a lapse in the discipline, you may well end up as the lion's lunch. However, if you put on a good show, permitting the lion to growl a bit and express its feelings, and if you move the act along to a satisfactory conclusion . . . then both you and the lion can honorably retreat to your separate quarters, satisfied that you performed well together and got the job done. But don't be fooled. You didn't reform the lion, you merely trained it how to act in an orderly manner for a predetermined purpose. Tomorrow, you will have to go back into the cage and repeat the whole performance with either the same or a different lion."

But whether the physician who doesn't want to share any part of what he sees as his responsibility is a lion or a lamb, it helps to know something about his background, what he wants out of life, and what are his principal satisfactions and frustrations. Cadmus has something to say about these and other circumstances influencing physician behavior, and some suggestions for effective response by administrators and trustees, including some useful tips about the questions that can be asked to elicit the kind of medical information needed for sensible planning without overstepping into the kind that physicians consider intrusive. Using right techniques, he is convinced, administrators and trustees can get physicians involved and helping with cost containment programs. What is needed is street sense. Not all of us have come down from the emotional high of the expansive years, Cadmus warns. "Not everybody's feet are on the ground. We look at things in the manner in which we were brought up, and we were brought up in a pretty expansive environment. Perhaps we are out of touch with reality. Perhaps there is some street sense we have missed. Those who can read the handwriting on the wall have sensed the coming of a new day. They have accepted the fact that they will have to keep their institutions alive with a lower census, with a tighter control on costs, and with an eye out for inter-hospital cooperation." Citing the case of a Milwaukee hospital that has a respected physician as a medical cost ombudsman, Cadmus concludes that "cost containment can't get to first base without the complete involvement of the entire medical staff . . . If it's done by a respected physician there will be no deterioration in the quality of care. So let's get on with it."

But it isn't that easy, and it may take more than street sense and ombudsmen, however respected. The physician's attitude toward cost may have been influenced by the expansive environment that is now vanishing, but its roots lie deep in the medical zeitgeist, where generations of physicians have believed that nothing but the best is worth having, and expense is no object. As the author of another new book for hospital trustees has it, "The budding physician is taught that cost is not *secondary,* but *unimportant.* What is important is solving the patient's problem, whatever it takes. That is part of the subtle curriculum." The subtle curriculum, Richard E. Thompson, M.D., explains, is the subtle effect of the educational experience on the student's attitudes and value system.[2] "The individual is usually unaware of these effects, even though they have an impact as great as the accumulation of specific academic knowledge, because they make him think and act in certain ways," says Thompson, an educational consultant for hospital boards and medical staffs who practiced medicine and taught medical students for several years before he became a consultant. Thus it is natural that doctors have been suspicious of cost containment, "because something from way back tells them that this emphasis will adversely affect their ability to obtain optimal results for patients. In fact, in their view, any person who would suggest that cost of care should be considered *at all* is probably completely out of touch with the realities of clinical practice."

Given this circumstance, communication, and even language, are important, Thompson suggests. Thus the physician for whom the words "cost containment" may evoke an image of meager resources, if not cut corners, might be perfectly comfortable with the concept of "cost-effectiveness," which considers cost in the context of acceptable care. In fact, communication and language are important not just for cost containment but in every aspect of the doctor-hospital relationship, which doesn't have to be as adversarial as it often is—in part because we live in a society that maximizes conflict disguised as socially acceptable competition and makes pushers and shovers of us all. Whichever way he looks today the physician sees a lurking adversary: Hospitals are gaining on him with more and more controls; government agencies and insurance companies demand mountains of paperwork; nurses want to take over his procedures and prerogatives; press and television spread suspicion and criticism instead of the esteem he anticipated; and even patients have to be seen as potential opponents in court. The instinctive response is resistance, and more often than not it focuses on the hospital, where his medical school teachers had led him to believe he would be "not only captain of the ship but owner of the line," as Thompson explains it. "He expected that walls would crumple when he blew his trumpet. In fact, some green administrator has the audacity to suggest that he is playing off key!"

Under the circumstances, trustees who think the way to deal with doctors is to take a hard line and show them who's in charge will almost certainly get the kind of confrontation they're looking for. Because they have the authority they can always win the battle—and prolong a war that can have only losers. Instead, Thompson thinks trustees should use their authority to mediate disputes and enhance institutional harmony. "In your position you can insist that groups vying for control can work out ways to share control, take new approaches to relieve the pressure-resistance cycle, and return to attitudes of professionalism and concern for the patient," he says. "Conflict and change are part of life, so a cooperative relationship does not mean that you will always avoid conflict and confrontation. But rediscovery of approaches other than an adversarial stance can minimize conflict and accomplish mutually beneficial results."

Thompson's suggestions for the rediscovery of other than adversarial approaches add up to a medical environment's adaptation of Dale Carnegie and the *New Testament,* combining the soft answer and turning the other cheek, but for those who may be scornful he has some examples suggesting that "It's my fault," and "Let me do that for you," and "I don't know"—words that are not heard every day in hospital corridors—may open a lot of doors that are often slammed in anger. Obviously, though understandably it isn't emphasized as much by Thompson, a physician, as it is by Cadmus, an administrator, the key actor in determining whether the institution emerges as an integrated organization or a collection of contending fiefdoms is the administrator. Cadmus sees him as a leader who motivates rather than commands. "Exercising leadership is not unlike being good parents to teenagers," he said. "You can't order, you can't lecture, you have to share power and turn things in a constructive direction—and then hope for the best." With an eye for detail, Cadmus also suggests that an administrator is likely, if not certain, to be a more effective motivator if his desk is clean, his pants are pressed, and he gets to meetings on time.

Like Cadmus, Thompson thinks we aren't going to get anywhere by insisting on an answer to the question about who's running this place. "The question, 'Who's in charge?' asks you to decide whose claim to absolute control is best justified," he says. "This only stimulates power struggles. On the other hand, the question, 'In charge of what?' asks you to better understand the hospital's component functions and may suggest the checks and balances model of governance. The individual physician remains the primary decision maker in the context of caring for an individual patient. In that context, he is entitled to expect hospital personnel to respond to his direction . . . The administrator should be able to concede the individual physician's prerogatives as long as the doctor doesn't try to invade the administrator's sphere of control," Thompson is willing to say that the administrator is the chief operations officer of the hospital in the same way the president is the chief operations officer of the corporation, but his concept of checks and balances clearly considers that full authority over the medical staff resides with the board, not the executive. "The corporate structure concept has led some management professionals to think that their responsiveness to the trustees is more important than their responsiveness to the medical staff," he concludes. "In fact, some administrators who have not understood the need to respond to both groups have been checked and balanced right out of the hospital."

The Thompson view of checks and balances isn't always clear, but his uneasiness about administrators as presidents makes itself felt. "Most administrators are good guys," he says at one point, "but occasionally it may be necessary for trustees and medical staffs to exercise their right to reject self-serving interpretations of the corporate structure concept." And again, "Unfortunately, in some hospitals the corporate structure brought with it not only the positive effects of sound business management but also the negative effects of cutthroat competition, including individual struggle for control." In some cases the formal training of recently graduated hospital administrators has tended to emphasize the medical staff as an adversary, Thompson suggests, and ". . . the CEO starts off on the wrong foot by explaining to the medical staff that the corporate bylaws put him in charge of everything, including the doctors. To the doctors, this may sound like a blatant power grab, and if they receive no explanation as to why a soundly run hospital needs a focal point for managerial responsibility, they withdraw to their lounge to sulk and plot the revolution."

Wherever he graduated, a CEO who starts off by explaining that he is in charge of the doctors is not only on the wrong foot but in the wrong business, and it seems doubtful that anybody with brains enough to cope with today's rigorous training of hospital administrators could be so lacking in common sense. Such lapses have to be explained by the fact that superior brains sometimes reside in.overweening egos; the combination may be accommodated in the university environment and is not unsuited to success in the professions, but it is incompatible with the demands of administration, which puts a premium on resiliency and rewards patience more than pride. So it doesn't matter much in the end whether the title is president or administrator, or whether the organizational construct is corporate or traditional not-for-profit. What does matter is that everybody on the premises should understand who does what. The answer to "Who runs this place?" might be anything from a czar to a town meeting, as long as everybody knows how the system works. That isn't what either Cadmus or Thompson had in mind, but whoever is running the place can learn a lot from both of them about how it works, or why it doesn't.

[1]Cadmus, R.R., Hospitals Are Us, Chicago: Teach'em, Inc., 1979, p. 183.

[2]Thompson, R.E., Helping Hospital Trustees Understand Physicians, Chicago: American Hospital Association, 1979, p. 82.

The Way We Were— and Are

February 1980

One of the most forward-looking persons I have ever known, a man whose bright vision of the future cheered and illuminated the lives of all his friends and associates, was nearing 80 when I was half that old, and he used to warn me that if I ever got to the place where I thought everything was better in the old days I should keep quiet about it, or risk boring everybody to death—including myself. So I am a little timid about embarking on this exercise of then-and-now, lest it should have that unhappy result. But I rationalize that there are a few things, always, that we can learn from the past, and anyway, one's view of the world is as much a product of his genes as of his age. Besides, keeping a bright vision of the future, the way things are going, has got to be a lot harder work now than it was 30 years ago.

What I was doing 30 years ago was mostly reporting hospital affairs, which is mostly what I do now—a circumstance that could mean either that I am an unusual constant in an unstable world or that I am in an awful rut. Either way, it presents me with an opportunity to make some comparisons of what hospital trustees and administrators and physicians worked at and worried about, then and now. What trustees worked at for the most part 30 years ago was raising money and building additions, and what they worried about, in addition to maintaining a prudent relationship between revenue and expense, was the fact that management of their growing institutions was entrusted to a person who didn't look like or talk like a businessman or, if he had been to one of the new university graduate programs in hospital administration, seemed too young to be in charge of what was becoming a large-scale business. But then, trustees comforted one another, it wasn't really a business, was it?

The trustees in those days didn't worry much about patient care. That was the doctors' affair. The more advanced hospitals had what they called joint conference committees whose trustee and medical staff representatives got together regularly to assure one another that everything was under control, just the way the American College of Surgeons hospital standardization program said it should be. There may have been an occasional grumble from doctors who thought hospital contracts with radiologists and pathologists amounted to the corporate practice of medicine, which was unlawful. But the more common view was that this was just trouble being stirred up by the specialists' societies, and it would go away. As a matter of fact, the issue got even more troublesome later on and never did go away; it simply got lost among the greater complexities that arose when the courts started deciding that trustees are responsible not just for doctors on contract but for all doctors. Wherever they may have got to, those trustees of a generation ago would be astonished if they could sit in on a board or committee meeting today when a matter of staff credentials is under consideration, or when trustees are reviewing medical statistics and asking questions about staff performance. They're still a little shy about it, but they understand that the doctors' business is their business too.

Old-time trustees would be horrified, also, if they were to review a current hospital financial statement and identify the revenues coming from the government programs. "Why, that's socialized medicine!" they would expostulate. So it is, if you want to call it that, and today's trustees spend a measurable share of their time helping the management devise means of conforming to and coping with the rules and standards their trustee forebears always knew would result if government entitlements to medical care should ever be enacted.

Without the perplexities of quality assurance and government intervention, how did the trustees of those earlier, easier days spend their time? It would be foolhardy to suggest that the report of a single hospital board meeting 30 years ago could be considered typical of anything but itself, but for what it is worth a report that has come to hand indicated that the board handled without comment reports on current operations and fund raising, discussed and decided on a room rate increase but held back approval of an increase in service charges, rejected out of hand a proposal that selected department heads should attend board meetings other than by specific invitation to discuss particular problems, and apparently spent the greater part of the meeting discussing a dispute involving the OR supervisor and a surgeon who was obviously competent and productive, but intransigent. It was the kind of problem that would be resolved now if not by an assistant then surely by the chief administrator, and would be brought to the attention of the board only if it resulted in either lawsuit or assassination.

With the exception of the rare trustee who was either retired or fanatic in devotion to the hospital, or both, and spent most of his time there masterminding everything that went on, board members in the old days generally gave it an hour or two a month for a meeting and maybe another hour or so for a committee assignment, if there was one, and a little more than that for a few weeks every few years during a fund-raising drive. There are still some fanatics, and some dilettantes, around today, but the rule for trustees now is a lot less meddling in management by the overzealous and a lot more time studying and attending meetings and taking part in the discussions and decisions. In contrast to their predecessors, trustees are aware that they are accountable to somebody besides themselves, though they aren't very clear about just who else it is, and neither is anybody else. Depending on what the decisions have to do with, accountability today slips in and out of focus like a television picture in a high rise, and the only thing trustees can be sure of is that it isn't just us. Who it is depends on what it is.

The then-and-now difference in administrators is not only in what they do but also in who they are. Yesterday's roster was a grab bag: physicians who were either retired or weaned from practice, including many who as chief residents discovered a talent and liking for administration; up-from-the-ranks nursing superintendents and accountants who grew into or fell into chief administrator appointments and got the job done as long as they saluted in the halls—and no longer; clergy and religious whose dedication to mission may have outrun their experience on occasion without anybody noticing, and the then-new products of the budding university programs, including all the above but more often young, bright, ambitious, and inexperienced, not the saluting type but with a tendency to last longer if they knew when to go through the motions. Whoever they were, their jobs were complicated and demanding, but they would be regarded as elementary by today's executives, who dash from meeting to meeting throughout the day and half the night encountering a wild variety of adversaries and allies and drawing on an extraordinary stockpile of knowledge and experience, constantly negotiating and always knowing that success, for themselves and their institutions, may depend more than anything else on judging when to compromise and when to stand firm. Solomon should live so long.

There are still some physicians and up-from-the-ranks achievers, and religious, running hospitals this way, and they have to be good at it to survive. But the prevailing mode today is the type that was trained for the job, and the key to his view of the assignment is that he wants to be, and be known as, president or chief executive officer, or both. The word administrator is considered somehow belittling, probably because it doesn't convey quite the desired image of man in charge. And today's hospital, like today's society, values image as much as substance. In some ways, things *were* better in the old days.

In any case, the chief executive today is innundated with data and surrounded by assistants. These supports unquestionably make management more efficient than it was before computers and make it possible, at least, for managers to keep abreast of the complexities emerging from the proliferation of specialization, technology, and regulation and the opacities resulting from changing reimbursement practice. But the biggest change of all from the linear administration of a past generation may be in the extent to which the focus of executive attention lies outside rather than inside the hospital. That's where the action is today. If you see a chief executive in a patient's room, you can be confident that he is (a) in a small or church-owned institution, (b) dropping in on a friend, or (c) over 60.

All this is not to say that administrators, or presidents, aren't interested in patient care. They are, and they have computer printouts on their desks to prove it. To a degree that yesterday's administrators would have considered impossible, patient care has become something that a statistic, or at any rate a collection of statistics, can measure, and, after a fashion, evaluate. The president can sit in his office reading printouts and make a judgment of how well the hospital is doing its job that is probably a lot more accurate than any impression he might get from prowling the halls asking patients "How's everything?" Thus the efficient manager and board of trustees can put patient care in the aggregate on the scale and weigh it, along with finance and plant operations and the latest public opinion poll, and keep a score of hospital performance—something trustees and administrators in the past had to do by some combination of observation and guesswork.

Computers measure patient care in the aggregate, however, and patients are cared for one at a time by physicians, nurses, and others, and the difference betweeen the collective and distributive values in patient care is what causes a large share of the problems that can arise among hospitals and their doctors. The different perspectives have always been there, but they didn't cause so many problems in the days of laissez-faire boards that weren't accountable to government agencies for their collective statistics and to courts for their distributive results, which are the primary responsibility of physicians. Thus it has been changing external circumstance, and not any wish to intervene, much less dominate, that has compelled trustees and administrators to introduce systems for seeing that patient care is monitored and to concern themselves with matters their predecessors for the most part peacefully ignored. The coming together of doctors and hospitals has been altogether necessary, if not altogether happy.

Actually, it isn't altogether, either. Doctors on hospital boards and on board and management committees have still got a way to go to be effective, and trustees and administrators on medical staff committees are still so new as to be stiff and a little uncomfortable, like new shoes. But they will get broken in, because the direction is irreversible. In the old days, trustees, administrators, and physicians used to talk piously about the three-legged stool and tell one another what a strong structure it was. That was good enough at a time when the trustees got the money and the doctors got the patients and the administrator got them out of each other's way, and all they had in common was a roof. But one leg or another, or all three, could break down under today's pressures.

What is required instead is a solid structure, and that is the reason so many hospitals have been adopting what has been described as the corporate form of organization. However, the way it is being done often leaves the doctors on the outside wondering what's going on inside, and that won't work either. The hospital today needs the adaptability and maneuverability that the corporate form of organization affords, but unless it comprehends physicians as part of the organizational structure, it will risk losing sight of what it is adapting and maneuvering for. Those trustees who used to worry because the hospital was a business that wasn't wholly a business knew what they were worrying about. It still isn't.

Get All the Working Parts Together

November 1980

"I took on this job because I realized somebody had to do it, and I thought it might be fun," a hospital trustee remarked at a trustees' conference not long ago. "Now the government is telling us we can't build the addition we were counting on, the doctors tell us they don't need the kind of evaluation studies the Joint Commission tells us they have to do, the hourly paid employees have joined a union we didn't want, and a court has just ruled against us in a malpractice case. I thought it was going to be fun, but not this much fun."

Everybody laughed, but only because hospital trustees are too old to cry. After the meeting, this trustee was asked if he had really considered that it was going to be fun to be on the hospital board. He thought a minute and said, "I suppose fun isn't the right word. But I did think it would be satisfying to work with a group of good people for an institution we're proud to represent and we all know is needed. And it has been satisfying, in a way, but also frustrating." Why frustrating? So many problems? "That, of course. But there are always problems, everywhere. You expect that. The frustrating thing is that the conditions keep changing, so we can't have any confidence that the solutions we work out today will be any good tomorrow."

In a society that will be pleased if the inflation drops to 10 percent and the embarrassments of a national election can be relieved, if not forgotten, confidence that today's solutions will be any good tomorrow may be too much to expect for any business or occupation, but it does seem that for the past few years the hospital business has outdistanced most others in its rate of change. This is a circumstance that probably results more than anything else from the fact that the entire complex or system of professional services was transformed overnight from wholly private to largely public accountability by the enactment of public entitlements amounting to nearly half of its

283

total activity. That happened only 15 years ago, and most of the changes and problems of these years—fiscal, professional, and managerial—have to do with making public accountability work in a private system. Many private industries have some public accountabilities, to be sure, but for the most part these are well established, having been developed over the years in large, highly organized corporations, as in the utilities and transportation industries. In contrast, public accountability came all at once to the hospital field, and nobody on either the public or private side knew how to make it work in a professional service culture consisting of small, independent institutions and individual practitioners. The learning process has been painful for everybody as the rules and conditions have kept changing, especially because the changes are determined as much by political and bureaucratic maneuvering as by anybody's judgment of what works and what doesn't.

Trying to work within the rules and make the rules work, hospital trustees and executives and physicians spent a large part of their time during the last half of the 1970s in activities having to do with planning, and it may be instructive now to consider how this came about and what has happened. Beginning immediately after the public entitlements were enacted, or as soon afterward as the Medicare and Medicaid bills started coming in, the Congress sought to achieve economies in the provision of these services by encouraging cooperative planning and sharing of facilities and services. In rapid succession the Comprehensive Health Planning, Partnership for Health, and Regional Medical Program acts were passed, and bureaus were established in the Department of Health, Education and Welfare to help hospitals that had always competed vigorously for physicians and patients and excellence and prestige to curb their competitive instincts and learn to love and share with their neighbors. Some trustees and executives did indeed start to talk to and meet with other boards and administrators, and some sharing of plans resulted. But the competition continued unabated, and the bills went up instead of down. So when the lawmakers passed the Social Security Amendments of 1972, they included section 1122, which said in effect, "Love and share with your neighbors, *damn it!*"

That got a little more action. More states got certificate-of-need laws; hospital trustees and executives served on planning agency boards and went to planning agency meetings; some shared service arrangements came to mean not just purchasing and laundry and data processing but "you take the obstetrics and pediatrics and we'll take the long-term care," and that got the doctors into the act. But the competition and the inflation went right on anyway, and in 1974 the Congress passed the National Health Planning and Resources Development Act, creating a whole national planning apparatus with authority to say who does what. It doesn't always stick, but it hurts a lot even when it doesn't, so that produced more action still. But it wasn't all exactly what the planners had in mind. Trustees and executives and doctors spend a lot of their time now on planning matters, some of it considering what the neighbors are doing and fitting their services and plans to regional needs accordingly, but probably a lot more of it figuring how they can beat the neighbors out of planning authority approval for a particular equipment or facility improvement.

Another kind of action that has resulted from the planning act is the rapid organization—one might say flight—of independent hospitals into multihospital systems, and these haven't turned out to be just what the planners envisioned either. What they had in mind was what health care planners have always had in mind—neat regional systems of referral linkages from outpatient stations to small rural or neighborhood hospitals to larger community hospitals and on to the great academic medical centers. The planners call these vertical systems, and a few of them, or parts of a few of them, have emerged. But most of the systems operate to effect some consolidation of management services, and it is hoped some economies, and some improvement in the clinical services that are already there, and perhaps eventually some consolidation and regionalization of the clinical services. This would be possible in only a few of the systems at best, however, because most of them ignore geographic considerations entirely; in most cases hospitals across the street from each other or a few blocks apart would rather belong to separate systems and keep on competing. And in any event if you asked a trustee—any trustee—to testify under oath about the reasons his hospital joined a system, the answer you'd get from most of them would be, "So we could deal more effectively with the HSA, the PSRO, third parties, rate reviewers, and legislators." That isn't bad, but it does suggest that to some extent the system works to beat the system.

Neither trustees nor executives nor physicians are unaware that the purpose of the whole regulatory effort has been to contain costs, and since it has obviously been impossible to keep costs from rising in a wildly inflationary period, the scapegoating that resulted has singled out the hospital system as inefficient, and further reforms now appear inevitable. It seems likely that the next turn of the wheel, with some new spinners on the job, will bring us another wholly new set of laws and regulations. Laid on hospitals whose competitive activities have been restrained by most of the laws and regulations of the past 15 years, the new laws and rules are being proposed and will be introduced as measures that are needed to make hospitals more competitive. This is something like stepping on the brake and the accelerator at the same time and seems wasteful of both muscle and energy, but if it's going to happen that way, the hospitals best prepared to deal with the consequences will be those whose trustees, administrators, and physicians have learned how to work together more closely in meeting the planning, quality control, and cost containment crises of the past five years than they had commonly done in easier times. In those hospitals, the boundaries of the old territorial jurisdictions—money, management, and medicine—have become blurred, and the walls between them have crumbled. Some trustees are deeply involved in planning, and some in management, and some in quality assessment. Administrators take part in formulating policies in all these areas. Physicians no longer turn pale or purple when trustees or administrators ask questions about medical care, nor do physicians refrain from asking questions about money and management. There are lines still that haven't been breached, and won't be, and shouldn't be. Trustees and administrators don't tell doctors what to do, or not do, for individual patients; doctors don't tell executives how to conduct meetings or negotiate contracts; administrators don't tell the finance committee of the board how to invest endowments. But they all know a lot about one another's business and responsibilities, and they don't hesitate to make suggestions, or listen to them.

In contrast, places that have kept the old boundaries intact, with trustees, administrators, and doctors nodding politely at meetings and going their separate ways, seem certain to lose out if the new turn of the wheel should indeed bring on, as some are insisting should be the case, an era of price competition that will have hospitals bidding against one another for contracts with HMOs, employed groups, and whatever kinds of promoters' schemes the new law and its regulations won't succeed in excluding. Economists and other critics of traditional hospital methods have been talking glibly about all the economies and efficiencies that will flow when hospitals are forced to "maintain a competitive position in the marketplace," as they say, making the whole thing sound like a Turkish bazaar. It probably won't get quite that raffish, but it is possible that in coming years competition could reach the point where hospitals will be called on to make fast, and right, decisions or risk losing patients or money, or both. If that happens, institutions with clearly established lines of authority and responsibility, including physicians at top levels of governance and management, will be in the best positions to make judgments and respond to changing competitive circumstances. The board of trustees that has to wait around while the doctors hold a series of town meetings to decide whether or not they want to participate in a capitation plan, for example, isn't going to get the chance to find out whether it would work or not. In any instance that might be the result the doctors want—until the hospital goes broke.

Of course, these are caricatures. The well-organized hospitals are not really that coherent, and the poorly organized hospitals are not that chaotic, and the market for medical services is not going to become an auction. Practices and values and modes of thought that have been developed over generations and have worked well for most of the population are not that easily overturned. The cost problem that is the reason for the cry for reform exists throughout the economy, not just in medical services, and the proposed solution, price competition, wouldn't work anyway, because the market for medical services is peculiarly insensitive to price. Buyers of medical services, including corporate buyers, care less about price and more about safety and quality and continuity and convenience, and these values would be threatened, not protected, by the proposed reforms.

But the political appeal of reform, and especially of this reform at this time, is formidable, and some response is probably inevitable, and whatever it turns out to be, it will still be true that the hospitals with the most coherent organization of decision-making authority are the ones most likely to cope successfully with change. Wherever an institution may find itself along the organizational scale from chaos to coherence, the direction to take will be clear as soon as the goal is clear, and the goal is simple: get all the working parts together. It's a lot easier to say than it is to do, given the organizational tradition that identified a board of trustees, an administration, and a medical staff as separate entities and rarely considered that they usually were entities within a single hospital corporation. And even when medical staffs were incorporated separately, as some were at times when fears of "hospital domination" obtruded, they were still separate corporations within a single hospital structure; a medical staff doesn't float around in space attached to nothing. Under any circumstances, coherence isn't achieved by organization charts; the tidiest charts often bear little resemblance to the way an organization works, but all those hospital organization charts that show an orderly hierarchy of authority from the board through the administrator to all the departments, with a dotted line shooting off sideways to the medical staff, may reflect exactly what is happening, because what a dotted line on an organization chart actually means is, "We don't really know how this is supposed to work."

How is it? Whatever the chart shows, it isn't going to work very well if the doctors are off there by themselves without taking part in any of the activities subsumed in the organization, because that's where they do their work, and their work is what the organization is there for. Something may be accomplished by changing the bylaws to make the board of trustees a board of directors and making the chief administrator a member of the board and calling him president or chief executive officer, if that's what he really is, instead of administrator. But this by itself won't achieve coherence, and neither will coherence be improved, and it may be damaged, by just erasing the dotted line and pulling the medical staff in as a department under the board and the president, because no matter how it looks on the chart, the medical staff obviously isn't just another department, and the doctors are likely to be disaffected, if not infuriated, by any implication that this is the case.

Looking around at the way boards and administrators work with doctors in what appear to be successfully integrated institutions, one can quickly conclude that there isn't any one right way to do it. Some make the relationship work by having doctors on all the principal board and management committees and board members on medical staff committees, with administrators providing support service or, as they like to say, "liaising" all over the place. Others remain traditionally detached, dotted lines and all, but manage by effective communications up and down the line to keep doctors informed and involved in the big decisions. When they are clued in all along and understand the pressures of cost containment and regulatory requirements and reimbursement constraints and, coming if not already present, strong competitive interests, physicians view hospital financial security and survival the same way trustees and administrators do. Physicians who see the hospital as an adversary and take their positions accordingly do so because they have been conditioned to see it that way by trustees and administrators who think doctors can't possibly understand finance. The obverse side of that, naturally, is, "Laymen can't possibly understand patient care." When these positions become ankylosed, as they often do, real communication ceases. Messages may be sent, but they are not received. "The doctors get our operating and financial statements," trustees and administrators say. "The trouble is they don't read them." Under those circumstances, they never will.

In the end, the coherent institution is the result more of attitudes than of techniques. But in most hospitals, even those where the adversarial mode has prevailed for years, there are one or two trustees, at least, and one or two physicians, who have come to understand that the external pressures of the years ahead could destroy a place that is not together enough to respond to changes in the environment, whether these come in the form of new laws and regulations, changes in reimbursement practice, new methods of delivering care, new alliances with hospital systems, or competition with other institutions. The task of these few trustees and physicians then becomes the difficult one of changing the attitudes of their associates—if necessary, one at a time. The process is already under way in many institutions. It began some years ago in most places with the election of physicians to the boards of trustees. To make it more than an empty gesture, this needs to be followed by the appointment of physicians to board and management committees, the involvement of physicians in financial and management decisions, the reformation or phasing out of "anti-doctor" administrators, the appointment of trustees to medical staff committees, and, always, the continuing, conscientious, systematic effort to communicate.

The communications effort is the most important of all these, and in many cases it may be the only thing that can be done right away, because in ankylosed hospitals neither doctors nor trustees are ready to trust one another to the point where the exchange of committee appointments would be either possible or effective. For the same reason, formal reports or other printed communications are not likely to accomplish much in these hospitals either, until the ground has been prepared by means of a carefully planned program of conversations and meetings. These begin with the leaders who are already disposed toward amicable understanding. In embedded adversarial situations, the conversations may have to proceed gradually from physician to physician and trustee to trustee, aimed at testing and modifying attitudes, and then move on to meetings where all the problems and pitfalls and opportunities are laid out and all the questions discussed. This is where leadership counts: without it, meetings can be disastrous. But with knowledgeable, patient, and wise leadership—and this might be provided by a trustee, or a physician, or an administrator—such meetings or series of meetings can go a long way toward dissipating mistrust and bringing an institution to a position of readiness to respond to the pressures of the 1980s.

With appropriateness review bearing down, and HCFA's diagnostic-related group reimbursement already in prospect, and HMOs cranking up all over the landscape, and price competition now apparently being sold to the Congress as the panacea for all the cost problems of the health care system, the '80s are not going to be a cakewalk for anybody. But the hospital that is prepared, or getting prepared, for all these and whatever other vicissitudes are waiting in the wings, the hospital with a governing board, an administrative staff, and a physician group that are meeting and talking and thinking together is likely to survive the decade intact. And the larger the number of such coherent, responsive hospital organizations, the better the chances that 1990 will see a health care system that looks a lot like the health care system of 1980 and is meeting the needs of the population by action that is still largely voluntary.

Systems: Good News
and Bad News

August 1980

What may readily be the greatest change in American hospitals since Ben Franklin and Thomas Bond got their heads together in Philadelphia in 1751 has been the recent movement of institutions into arrangements with one another varying all the way from a shared scanner to a nationwide conglomerate. Whatever they are, the arrangements have all been described and evaluated in an extraordinary outpouring of books and articles on the subject published over the past 10 years, and especially the past five years that have seen so much activity in the formation and expansion of multihospital management systems, as the more binding agreements are commonly called. The evaluations offer a mixed bag of conclusions. It is obviously difficult, and perhaps misleading, to generalize about a decade of experience during which change has been so rapid, but it seems clear that the promised economies that have been the ostensible lure of the systems have been realized only slowly in some cases, and not at all in others. Where costs have gone up instead of down at rates suggesting that something more than inflation has been at work, the reason in most cases apparently has been that system start-up costs had been higher and start-up periods longer than anybody had foreseen would be the case, and that standards of patient care and management were being elevated in hospitals joining the systems, with the initial effect of adding rather than subtracting cost.

Another message that emerges unmistakably from even a cursory review of the literature is that operating a system isn't what anybody would call uncomplicated, and joining a system may create as many problems as it solves for the unit manager. The message is clear, if implicit, in a pair of titles appearing in a recently published bibliography on multihospital systems. The title of an article published in the early 1970s was typical of its time: "Prospects for Efficiencies and Economies Are Leading to Creation of Multihospital Organizations," this said. And a 1979 title suggests the complexities of the decade: "Legal and Financial Constraints on the Development and Growth of Multiple Hospital Arrangements."

However severe the constraints, the point now is that the systems are better prepared to deal with them than their constituent units would have been by themselves, and it is probably this dependence on superior resources, more than any great passion for efficiency and economy, that has impelled the movement to management systems. Improvements in patient care and management efficiency will be realized over time and demonstrated in studies yet to come, without much question, but the basic motivation has been more safety than efficiency. The goal is survival, and this suggests that the systems will continue to grow no matter what, because the environmental threats to the freestanding hospital are not going to go away. Ultimately, what is at stake may be the survival of the voluntary structure of hospitals in an economy whose complexity tends to extinguish small enterprise—in health and education as it does in business and industry.

Actually, it is likely that there are as many specific reasons hospitals have been joining together in systems as there are hospitals joining systems, having to do for the most part with some aspect of finance, management, governance, operations, patient care, planning, or marketing, or all of these things. So to describe this plexus of motivations as either survival or efficiency, or both, is obviously simpleminded, but like many simpleminded propositions it may also be essentially true. When a governing board comes to consider the desirability of joining an organization or system whose resources in one way or another would afford a measure of security, or efficiency, or service that the institution itself cannot expect to achieve, it has to weigh these putative advantages against the possibility, at least, of offsetting losses. To what extent, for example, will the autonomy of the board itself give way to system authority in the proposed arrangement? Inevitably, there will be some who see any such affiliation as an invasion of community and institutional pride, and independence, and freedom to make choices. This is not a prohibitive barrier to action, but these are real values that have to be put on the scale and weighed. If some reorganization of the decision-making process at either the board or management level is contemplated, what consideration is to be given to the possible impact on the community, not to mention all the persons involved?

Often among the more sensitive of the circumstances requiring careful examination are those involving physicians. Some doctors may rejoice at the prospect of new opportunities in capital financing, with visions of splendid new facilities and equipment. But others may see new and remotely applied, and hard to get at, constraints on spending. Another situation that is not uncommon is one in which a community hospital is faced with fading occupancy and aging physicians, a combination that plainly calls for aggressive recruitment that the local doctors may not want and the local board is therefore reluctant to initiate. The new authority furnished by a management contract or multihospital system may provide a heaven-sent answer, but it isn't going to be easy for anybody—least of all for the newly recruited doctor or doctors when they arrive on the scene, and had better bring along some qualifications for sainthood, as well as professional certification. Obviously, if a situation of this kind results in the successful recruitment of qualified new physicians through use of system resources, and hence improved occupancy and restored fiscal health for the hospital, the community and everybody in it will benefit eventually, and the temporary pain for a few physicians and perhaps patients and others will be a small price to pay.

But the pain may be more lasting for some, especially where transfer of ownership or governing or management authority is involved and the effects can be expected to reverberate up and down the line, with winners and losers in every class from doctor to doorman. Under these circumstances, the impact on rank-and-file employees is the feeling of uncertainty about what is going to happen and the accompanying apprehension or nervousness about what it may mean. Conscientious boards and managers know, or should know, that such vibrations are inevitable, and in an effort to forestall fears and sustain morale they often prepare carefully worded messages stressing the positive aspects of the affiliation, whatever it is, and either omitting any mention of what it may mean to employees or assuring them that it means only added security and opportunity for everybody. The messages are printed in employee publications or distributed in special employee bulletins, and the management considers then that everything has been done that can be done, in view of the fact that all the operating details haven't been worked out yet and the bland generalities of the messages are really all that can be said.

The only trouble with this practice is that the messages in employee publications and bulletins either aren't read or aren't believed, and in either case they are no match for the rumors that are bound to arise in connection with any major organizational change. One of the benefits of affiliation with a system for the hospital with limited personnel resources should be the capability for assessment of employee attitudes and management policies, and a systematic approach to the solution of whatever communications difficulties may be revealed—including epidemic nervousness and the rumors it engenders.

As one would expect, the multihospital literature is well supplied with examples of the ways in which patient care is improved through affiliation with systems: enhanced capital and equipment resources, tested techniques for physician and nurse recruitment, higher standards for professional and technical personnel, enriched staffing, new referral and consulting opportunities, and others. But there may also be risks. One misgiving about the patient care implications of management systems is that when some decisions—about facilities and resources and money and personnel and standards—are in some part removed from the local institution to a more remote authority, some measure of responsibility may go with them, and when local pride and local initiative are diminished, however slightly, local vigilance and local concern may also be diminished accordingly. If there is a risk, it is mostly to the caring component of quality—the comforts, and amenities, and personal concern for patient's feelings as well as patients' records, the component that some hospital critics have said is already diminished by the onrushing specialization and technology and preoccupation with the business of hospitals, as opposed to the mission of hospitals.

Of course, the impersonalization of care need not be accelerated or aggravated by an institution's affiliation with a management system; where appreciation of the importance of the caring component and awareness of the risk exist, system management could become the means of promoting rather than suppressing the kind of concern that is seen as deteriorating in so many institutions today. But the odds are against it; the prevailing emphasis in management systems is management, and the prevailing emphasis in management today is cost-effectiveness, and caring and concern are not notably cost-effective except in a perspective that envisions the long-term future of the entire voluntary hospital enterprise, as well as next month's profit-and-loss statement.

In a recent interview, a well-known social critic talked about another industry that has been moving rapidly for the past several years from dispersion in relatively small, independent, locally owned and managed units into large corporate systems. "What I'm concerned with is that once they are in a big corporation they're forced to do certain things," he said. "They are among giants competing with each other, and the element of the competition is growth. . . . You have to grow in number of units, because then you've got lots of different properties and you're not so dependent on the ups and downs of one particular property. You do that by treating each of your properties as an accumulator of capital; each of your properties is a community enterprise, and each community enterprise has to contribute a given amount each year to the parent corporation. It used to have to do that to the independent owner too. But the owner lived in the community, had to deal with the community, and his future was in the community. If he chose to he could re-invest surplus profits back into the enterprise, back into the community. In a corporate chain, that cannot happen. A chain may improve the quality of the operation to a point where it will be less vulnerable, but only to a point where the corporation is protected. From then on they have a quota for sending money beyond their budget to the home office. And the home office is interested in investing that money elsewhere."[1]

That was Ben Bagdikian, and he was talking about the newspaper chains, which are rapidly draining the community influence out of what is essentially a community enterprise. Hospital people may dismiss his animadversions as irrelevant, and for the most part they may be right, but there is a feeling nevertheless that some of what he has described here is going on in the hospital field already, and there could be more unless this is seen as a danger not just to the caring component of patient services but to the voluntary community component of the hospital, and unless the caring component and the community component are valued as related phenomena that measure a large part of the difference between hospitals and, say, gas stations.

This can't be done by keeping hospitals out of chains, or management systems. Whether we like it or not, or whether it accomplishes all that has been envisioned for it or not, the movement of independent units into large systems is going to continue in the hospital field, as elsewhere, because this is the direction in which the entire society is moving. We've watched it happening for a generation or more in business and industry; it is well advanced in education as well as in health care. It is not going to be seriously resisted, and certainly not reversed, so the only thing to do is to welcome its benefits and do whatever can be done to modify its hurtful effects. In the society as a whole, as in hospitals, these have to do chiefly with the erosion of humanizing behavior in social transactions.

If something valuable is being sacrificed, why do we do it? It could be because most of us don't think something valuable *is* being sacrificed, or it could be because we're not aware of the loss until the value has been irretrievably damaged. But the basic reason is that we don't really have any choice. We are driven by the growth imperative of the social organism and the knowledge imperative of the human organism. We do it because we *can* do it; the knowledge imperative produces the technology, and the growth imperative demands its application. The wit who said recently that "If God wanted us to have these huge multinational corporations He'd have given us the brains to run them" had it precisely backwards. We have them *because* God gave us the brains to create the technology that made them possible and the need to grow that made them inevitable. The technology and the need to grow make multihospital systems inevitable, and we'll need all the help we can get to keep them humane.

[1]Johnson, P., Pressing Concerns, an Interview with Ben Bagdikian, The Reader, 9:1, April 18, 1980.

It's a Question of Ethics

December 1979

A seasoned administrator who was a recognized leader of hospital thought of his generation once explained that there isn't any right way to negotiate a hospital merger. "There are lots of wrong ways, however," he told a reporter who had asked what was probably a dumb question, "and one of them is to let everybody know what's going on and try to answer all the questions about services and facilities and jobs and practices while the terms are still being negotiated."

This executive had been a key actor in the consolidation of two major hospitals. The agreement to merge had been worked out by a small select committee representing the two boards of trustees, managements, and medical staffs, he said. When the committee had agreed on such major dispositions as name, governance, finances, and facilities, lawyers were called on to prepare detailed articles for review and action by the hospital boards creating the new entity. "When we announced the merger, it was an accomplished fact," he explained. That way, the people involved knew from the beginning that they had to live with it and make it work, and they did. The administrator was convinced that most of the questions about details of operations that would have delayed action and created confusion had simply disappeared, and those that remained had been resolved with less controversy and hardship than would inevitably have resulted if the process had been more open.

In the case of another merger, in another city, the open procedure had been followed. Here, for example, separate joint committees representing the medical staffs for each of some 20 specialty departments had met repeatedly to discuss details of the proposed arrangements. "They spent a whole year just arguing about beds," an administrator reported, "and it took them another year to reach any kind of consensus." But the ownership and management details had been simple by comparison, he related, "and the doctors could never say they weren't consulted."

In both these mergers, as in most of those that have been effected in the past 10 years, the boards of trustees of the merged hospitals were convinced that their actions were necessary to secure the future of their institutions and services, and that the results had been for the best interest of all the people concerned. It isn't by any means certain that all the doctors in both cases would agree, and it isn't possible on the evidence to state with certainty that the doctors who had been consulted were any better satisfied in the end than those who hadn't been. But assuming that there were no lasting ill effects in either case, it would appear that the first method was more efficient and generally preferable to the one that involved a year or more of argument and upset.

From the utilitarian point of view, this is obviously the case, but it can be argued that there may be an ethical question that isn't so easily settled. Is it right for a board of trustees to allow secret negotiations and take action affecting the lives of so many people without letting them know it is happening? Granted that neither the physicians nor the employees of the hospitals in any event could have been parties to the decisions, was there nevertheless a duty to let them know that the action was under consideration? Or was it rather a kindness, as well as an expedient, to spare them the prolonged uncertainties and apprehensions that would have occurred?

The utilitarian ethic rarely stands alone, and there may be other values that have to be considered, along with the fact that the merger was expedited by secrecy and it appeared that nobody lost any more than would have been the case no matter how it had been handled. If they had a choice, most people would prefer to know when their livelihoods are about to be subjected to the kind of scrutiny and manipulation that are inevitable for a certain number in any merger situation, and the failure to inform might thus be considered an injustice, if not an infringement of personal liberty—not for rank and file employees, perhaps, whose jobs in most cases would be unaffected, but for professional and management personnel at levels where the economies of merger are expected. In most hospital mergers, physicians on the active staffs retain their privileges at the merged institution, and in many cases the combined resources result in improved conditions of practice. But for some there may be disruptions such as changes in location or service that could cause inconvenience or expense, or perhaps loss of patients, and a strict sense of justice might imply a duty to warn of these possibilities.

In any merger, and perhaps in the one that has been referred to here, the decision makers on the boards and management staffs may weigh these ethical considerations conscientiously and still decide that on balance secrecy is justified, as it might be if it seemed likely that open discussion would actually jeopardize, and not just inconvenience, a conclusion that would plainly benefit more people than it could harm. Still another question that has to be weighed is the possibility that even with the most painstaking precautions, word of the negotiations may leak out, as often happens, in which case the responsible parties face an unpleasant choice between lying and acknowledging the truth, and in either case sacrificing the trust of those who may feel that they should have been informed.

If all these moral complexities obtrude in decisions for merger, consider how much more difficult the questions become when a hospital faces the possibility of having to shut down a facility or service, as economic or market pressures may require on occasion now, and as may happen with increasing frequency as the pressures continue in the future. For example, hospitals in many communities have been encouraged to close obstetric departments having consistently low occupancies; the departments are costly to operate and in the view of professional planners should be closed when patients can be referred to other hospitals within reasonable reach. In some cases, this has meant patients in labor must be transported 40 or 50 miles to have their babies, always at some cost of fear and inconvenience, and sometimes at hazard to the mothers and babies.

When such a move is proposed, what are the responsible trustees and administrators to think? The economic advantage to the hospital obviously has to be considered, and so does the fact that any saving the hospital may accomplish will mean some reduction in cost, however slight and indirect, to patients and other sources of payment. But the decision must also comprehend the impact on the patients and physicians and others who will be affected directly. How does one weigh a saving of, say, $100,000 a year for the hospital and the community against the anxieties of an unknown number of young families, and the putative hazard to an unknown number of unborn babies? Planners who recommend the consolidation of OB departments reject the notion that an hour's drive constitutes a real hazard and argue instead that only an OB department with several hundred births a year can furnish the quality of facilities and services that can safeguard the health of mothers and babies, and this is an argument that has to be taken seriously. May hospital decision makers say to themselves, "The planners recommend it, and there's nothing we can do about it"? Or do they have a moral obligation to resist the recommendation and continue the expense to protect those who would use the service? At what point is the balance of practical sense and abstract justice to be found? It is a distinguishing characteristic of hospital decision makers that not many of them would say flatly that either pragmatism or idealism should rule in every case, without consideration of the other—and this is something about hospitals that is commonly overlooked or unknown to their critics in government and business. There are business, professional, social, and moral values to be contemplated and judged in all important hospital decisions, and no computers or formulas to provide answers.

But there are some guiding principles that can help. One is the ideal of human behavior for centuries: Do unto others as you would they should do unto you. Not many of us behave according to the rule more than a fraction of the time; it seems likely that churches come closer to it than any other human institutions do, but surely hospitals are the only others that ever give it a thought. Bankers and lawyers and business executives who are hospital trustees are often criticized because "they leave their business brains outside the door when they enter the hospital boardroom," as the cliche has it. But it is to their everlasting credit that they do use an altogether different value system in the hospital boardroom, consulting their hospital hearts as well as their business brains. "How would I feel if this were done to me?" is not a question trustees commonly ask themselves in their offices downtown, and they would be looked at sideways if they did. But it can be a useful guide to hospital decisions; it won't put a dollar value on anxiety, but it can illuminate the need to consider the other values that are part of most hospital decisions.

Another rule that can often help is the first principle of medical ethics. The object of the profession, this says, is service to mankind, not personal gain. The ethic is as inescapably an unerring guide to right hospital decisions as it is to right physician behavior, and it is in no way diminished because there are hospitals, and physicians, who march to another tune. Obviously, personal gain is rarely a consideration in hospital actions. But institutional prestige or aggrandizement may be, and, when it calls for a different course from that prescribed by service, it is as wrong for the hospital as the fee for unneeded surgery is for the physician. No hospital can be expected to disregard a patient's ability to pay, or be paid for, but the ethic is understood instinctively by the public, and few circumstances are as damaging to public opinion of hospitals as are procedures that permit the inference that payment comes ahead of service, especially when an emergency, or perceived emergency, is involved.

There are ethics in business practice, and one of the principles is that the quality of the product must be consistent with its price. The purchaser of a cheap suit or coat doesn't expect that it will look as good or last as long as its higher priced equivalent would. He feels cheated when the product is inferior to what is expected at the price, but at most he has lost only the money, and he blames himself as much as he does the seller. When the product is a medical service, however, the ethical principle is an implicit guarantee of quality within the range of services offered. There is no such thing as a cheap or inferior medical service in the same sense that there may be cheap cars and cheap furniture. The patient who gets inferior service has been cheated at any price, and he may have lost a lot more than money. And the burden of blame is always on the provider, not the buyer or user, who has no basis for judging medical service as he judges suits and boots. Thus the limitation of services to those that can be offered with full assurance of their quality, and the maintenance of a system for assuring quality, are primary ethical responsibilities of hospital trustees and administrators and the physicians on their staffs. Medical care that is offered at a bargain is always suspect; the regulators and others who are seeking to inject massive doses of price competition into the market for medical services had better be certain that their schemes include some means of identifying the unethical institutions and practitioners that will be the first to promote their services to a public that trusts its doctors and hospitals and depends on an ethical standard that price competition could destroy. When the ethical standard is ignored or trimmed on occasion by doctors and hospitals, it is the considerable competition that already exists, as much as anything, that is responsible, and the kind of competition that economists and bureaucrats are so enchanted with now has often compelled basically decent businessmen to behave like predators. If it should force hospitals wholly into the competitive business mode, it might succeed in bringing down cost for some only by destroying value for everybody. The ethical standard that has been recognized for 2,500 years should be safeguarded, not scorned, by the society it benefits. Especially, it should be cherished by hospital trustees and administrators. As they face the hard decisions that confront them today, they will need all the business brains they can command, but the salvation of their institutions is the moral estate they have inherited.

INDEX

A

Aged,
    employment of, 146, 152-153,
      155
    graying of federal budget,
      147, 154
    health care of, 41-45, 148,
      160-162
    population projections,
      147-148
    poverty in, 145, 151
    retirement, 155
    as a social force 141-144, 149
    Social Security, 153
    (See also Medicare)

B

Blue Cross Association, 54-59

Bureaucracy, 91-95

Business ethic, 1-14
    corporate control of
      hospitals, 1-3
    industry vs. profession,
      205-208
    multi-hospital organization,
      10
    quality of patient care, 6-8

C

Clayton Act, 2

Competition, 18, 203, 240
    effect on quality of health
      care, 11-12, 75-76
    (See also Government
      regulation)

Consumerism, 21-24, 134-140
    community committees,
      136-137
    growth of consumer
      organizations, 138
    HSA boards, 137
    role of government, 139
    (See also Representative
      government)

Cost containment, 72, 244, 272
    and industry involvement,
      96-102
    public opinion, 103-104,
      176-197

E

Employee dissatisfaction,
    235-238